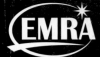

EMRA
Antibiotic Guide

16th Edition

Brian J. Levine, MD, FACEP
Editor-in-Chief

Christiana Care Health System
Department of Emergency Medicine

NOTICE

EMRA

Cathey B. Wise
Executive Director

Leah Stefanini
Meetings & Advertising Manager

Linda Baker
Marketing & Communications Manager

Rachel Donihoo
Publications & Communications Coordinator

Chalyce Bland
Administrative Coordinator

Disclaimer

This handbook is intended as a general guide to therapy only. While the editors have taken reasonable measures to ensure the accuracy of drug and dosing information used in this guide, the user is encouraged to consult other resources or consultants when necessary to confirm appropriate therapy, side effects, interactions, and contraindications. The publisher, authors, editors, and sponsoring organizations specifically disclaim any liability for any omissions or errors found in this handbook, for appropriate use, or treatment errors. Furthermore, although this handbook is as comprehensive as possible, the vast differences in emergency practice settings may necessitate treatment approaches other than presented here.

2015 EMRA ANTIBIOTIC GUIDE EDITORS

Editor-in-Chief

Brian J. Levine, MD, FACEP
Program Director
Emergency Medicine Residency Program
Department of Emergency Medicine
Christiana Care Health Services
Newark, DE
Associate Professor of Emergency Medicine
Jefferson Medical College
Philadelphia, PA

Senior Editors

Jamie Rosini, PharmD, BCPS
Joseph Romano, MD
J. Daniel Hess, MD
Brian A. Robertson, MD
Department of Emergency Medicine
Christiana Care Health System
Newark, DE

Nicole Srivastava, PharmD, BCPS
Christian Coletti, MD, FACEP
Stephen Boone, MD
Sherrill Mullenix

Authors

Faculty and Residents
Department of Emergency Medicine
Christiana Care Health System
Newark, DE

FOREWORD

It is a pleasure to present the new *2015 EMRA Antibiotic Guide*. Christiana Care's Emergency Medicine Residency Program is thrilled to provide this landmark publication for the *fifth time*!

Our goal has always been to create the easiest, quickest, most frequently utilized reference in the emergency department (ED). Based on extensive reader feedback, we have enhanced the content and ease-of-use even further. The new 2015 edition has been designed with simplicity in mind to maximize its utility in the fast-paced ED environment.

This endeavor was a year-long process involving the entire emergency medicine residency program at Christiana Care Health System. Each resident was asked to author a chapter or two, which were then diligently edited by our faculty attendings. This book would not have been possible without each physician's input.

The *EMRA Antibiotic Guide* is designed to be a quick-reference for antibiotic use only, not a text on the diagnosis or comprehensive treatment of disease. The content is color-coded and organized alphabetically by organ system, followed by sections on special topics to make reference quick and easy for each disease process. We have taken the Joint Commission's recommendations about avoiding medical errors one step further. Abbreviations have been eliminated where possible. For example, you will see "two times daily" as opposed to BID.

We also have attempted to simplify the sometimes-complicated pediatric dosing. Whenever possible, you will see the *individual* dosing for each medication that has a pediatric indication. Of special note, trimethoprim (found in TMP/SMX) dosing is based on the TMP composition. Weight-based dosing should be calculated on *actual* body weight unless otherwise noted.

In lieu of a standard antibiogram, which has been included in previous editions, we have decided that there is too much regional variation to comfortably trust a single chart. Instead, an antibiotic coverage table was designed. This table contains a listing of many common antibiotics from the book and the susceptibility of common organisms to each. In the current climate of increasing antibiotic resistance, this section will enable users to better tailor drug choices to target organisms. Residents will find this resource as valuable as the chapters themselves, but we caution that one should always consult local resistance data.

We are in an era where the bugs are gaining resistance faster than humans can develop antibiotics. One such organism, CA-MRSA (community-associated – methicillin-resistant *Staphylococcus aureus*) has altered our prescribing practice. We have addressed this issue, when necessary, to help avoid treatment failures.

The medications listed in this handbook are highly dependent on the editors' choices and may differ based on practice location. There may be other medications possible for individual indications that have been omitted. In cases where there are multiple antibiotic choices, we have chosen those that have the most data on efficacy or were least expensive. If the antibiotic choices were all considered equivalent, they were simply alphabetized. We have made every attempt to use specialty guidelines and peer-reviewed publications for each indication. It is our goal that every medication and dosage is as accurate as possible and we have made every attempt to avoid typographical errors (although they may occur). Patient condition should be taken into account with each antimicrobial prescribed. Alterations in dosing may be required for patients with renal or hepatic dysfunction.

We hope you find this guide helpful in the care of your patients during your daily practice. As always, EMRA encourages and appreciates your feedback. Thank you for making the *2015 EMRA Antibiotic Guide* a success!

— Brian J. Levine, MD, FACEP

ACKNOWLEDGEMENTS

The first edition of this book was conceived and edited by James D. Woodburn, MD, MS, and was published in cooperation with the Society of Academic Emergency Medicine (SAEM) in 1989-1990 under the title *EMRA Guide to Antibiotic Use in the Emergency Department*. The second edition, also published with the assistance of SAEM, was edited by Janet Williams, MD, and was published in 1991-1992.

The third edition in 1996 marked a turning point for this guide. James H. Bryan, MD, PhD, assumed the editorship. Dr. Bryan doubled the content of the book, changed the format, and took on the job of producing yearly updates to the text. Dr. Bryan remained an editor of this guide until the 2003 edition. His volunteer commitment to EMRA and this guide are unparalleled. Two others were integral to the editions edited by Dr. Bryan – Jon Jui, MD, MPH, and Barbara Bryan, PhD.

In addition, Greg Henry, MD, generously assisted in reviewing the first five editions of the book, and Kenneth Dirk, MD provided invaluable assistance with the major rewrites of the fourth, fifth, and sixth editions.

EMRA also thanks the many residents and faculty who have provided comments, criticisms, and suggestions for this guide. We are lucky to have physician assistants (PAs) and clinical pharmacists who work as part of our care team in the ED. Note that both the pharmacists and PAs are integral contributors to this edition. Our emergency- and infectious disease-trained pharmacists from Christiana Care (Jamie Rosini, PharmD, BCPS and Nicole Srivastava, PharmD, BCPS) continue to elevate each edition to another level. Special thanks to Casey M. Clements, M.D., Ph.D., assistant professor of emergency medicine at the Mayo Clinic for his peer-review for this edition. Also, special thanks to Sherrill Mullenix, executive assistant, Department of Emergency Medicine, Christiana Care Health System, for her invaluable assistance in the coordination and support of each edition. Ms. Mullenix has personally committed countless hours of review and coordination toward making this edition a success. Without Ms. Mullenix, this book would have been impossible to complete.

CONTRIBUTORS

All contributors are affiliated with Christiana Care Health System, Department of Emergency Medicine, Newark, DE, unless otherwise noted.

Editor-in-Chief
Brian J. Levine, MD

Authors
Eric Ahlers, MD
Gordon Reed, MD
  *Pelvic Inflammatory
  Disease
  Urethritis/Cervicitis*

Gina Ambrose, DO
Anuj Parikh, MD
  Cutaneous Abscess

Gina Ambrose, DO
Jason Nomura, MD
  Encephalitis

Saad Amin, MD
Paul Sierzenski, MD
  Pyelonephritis

Elise Attardo, DO
Richard Bounds, MD
  Pinworms

Elise Attardo, DO
Russell Queen, PA-C
  Thrush

Joel Atwood, MD
Stefanie Golebiewski-
Manchin, MD
  Open Fracture

Ilana Baltuch, MD
Patrick Matthews, MD
  *Necrotizing Fasciitis/
  Fournier's Gangrene*

Rachel Barney, MD
Angelo Grillo, MD
  Osteomyelitis

Rachel Barney, MD
Eli Zeserson, MD
  Botulism

Christopher Biedrzycki, MD
John Powell, MD
  Diabetic Ulcers

Christopher Biedrzycki, MD
Donnita Scott, MD
  Prostatitis

Stephen Boone, MD
Scott Edmondson, PA-C
  *Occupational Post-
  Exposure Prophylaxis*

Stephen Boone, MD
Gordon Reed, MD
  Bacterial Vaginosis

Lauren Brandltz, MD
Gordon Reed, MD
  *Sexual Assault
  Prophylaxis*

Diana Cer, DO
Christopher Giaquinto, PA-C
  Dental Abscess

Diana Cer, DO
Pamela Manzi, PA-C
  *Discitis/Vertebral
  Osteomyelitis*

Yin Chow, MD
Steve Kushner, MD
  *Septic Arthritis
  Septic Bursitis*

Valerie Cohen, DO
Robin Fitzgerald, PA-C
  *Acute Necrotizing
  Ulcerative Gingivitis*

Lauren Cooksey, MD
Julie Cooper, MD
  *Antibiotic Use
  During Pregnancy*

Lauren Cooksey, MD
Jason Nomura, MD
  *Pregnancy Class,
  Antibiotic Cost,
  Metabolism/
  Excretion Table*

Tam Dang, MD
Erin Watson, MD
  Ehrlichiosis

Andrew Deitchman, MD
Drew Pento, PA-C
  Neurocysticercosis

David Dinh, PharmD
Donnita Scott, MD
  UTI

Stephen Donnelly, MD
Christopher Rogan, MD
  Periorbital Cellulitis

Emily Emerich, MD
Robert Donovan, PA-C
  HSV

Ellen Finney, MD
Matthew Barrett, DO
  Pneumonia, Pediatric

Chesney Fowler-Lajczok, MD
Michael Diamond, PA-C
  Syphilis

Chesney Fowler-Lajczok, MD
Kathryn Groner, MD
  Epiglottitis

Emily Granitto, MD
Patrick Phelan, PA-C
Mammalian Bites

Michael Hansen, DO
Paul Krajewski, PA-C
Pharyngitis/Tonsillitis

Carolan Hass, MD
James Carroll, MD
Exacerbation of Chronic Bronchitis (AECB)

Carolan Hass, MD
William Paynter, PA-C
Malaria

Stephanie Hawley, MD
Patrick Phelan, PA-C
Rabies

J. Daniel Hess, MD
Jason Nace, MD
Antibiotic Coverage Table

Tamar Katz, MD
Christopher Cox, MD
Ludwig's Angina

Tamar Katz, MD
Erin Watson, MD
Intracranial Abscess

C. Elliot Lange, MD
Leo Burns, MD
Felon/Paronychia

C. Elliot Lange, MD
Julie Cooper, MD
Mastoiditis

Rosamund Lehmann, MD
Christian Coletti, MD
Parotitis/Sialoadenitis

Rosamund Lehmann, MD
John Madden, MD
Folliculitis

David Leventhal, MD
Tim Shiuh, MD
Pertussis

David Leventhal, MD
Pramod Vangeti, MD
Yersinia

Erica Locke, MD
Leila Getto, MD
Trichomonas

Erica Locke, MD
Stefanie Golebiewski-Manchin, MD
Candidiasis

Eleanore Maletta, MD
Walker Lee, MD
Tenosynovitis

Eleanore Maletta, MD
Jonathan McGhee, DO
Anthrax

Patricia Mangel, MD
Kathryn Groner, MD
Tetanus

Patricia Mangel, MD
Robert Rosenbaum, MD
Blepharitis

Vikram Marocha, MD
Kathryn Crowley, MD
Tinea Infections

Vikram Marocha, MD
Daniel Cummings, MD
Cryptococcus Neoformans

Timothy Medina, MD
Christopher Rogan, MD
CMV

Sean Morgan, MD
Patrick Matthews, MD
Orbital Cellulitis

Sean Morgan, MD
Jonathan McGhee, DO
Corneal Abrasion

Jeanhyong Park, MD
Blake Gustafson, MD
Smallpox

Jeanhyong Park, MD
Kristina Stransky, MD
Lice

Kenil Patel, MD
John Madden, MD
Cholangitis/Cholecystitis

Mark Pettit, MD
Walker Lee, MD
Diverticulitis/ Inflammatory Bowel Disease

Mark Pettit, MD
Jennifer Mink, MD
Tularemia

Kyle Plotts, MD
Jason Nace, MD
PCP

Kelly Potts-Eichhorn, MD
Dorothy Dixon, MD
Otitis Media

Kelly Potts-Eichhorn, MD
Jenna Fredette, MD
Otitis Externa

Maura Quinn, MD
Blake Gustafson, MD
Appendicitis

Maura Quinn, MD
Pramod Vangeti, MD
Meningitis

Vidya Raju, MD
Jennifer Mink, MD
Neutropenic Fever

7

CONTRIBUTORS

Nour Rifai, MBChB
Ross Megargel, DO
Toxoplasmosis

Nour Rifai, MBChB
Arayel Osborne, MD
Endocarditis

Brian Robertson, MD
Eric Felker, PA-C
Lyme

Brian Robertson, MD
Brent Passarello, MD
Cephalosporin Reference

Joseph Romano, MD
Ryan Arnold, MD
Sepsis

Novneet Sahu, MD
Theresa Nguyen, MD
*Adverse Reactions
and Drug Interactions*

Novneet Sahu, MD
Brent Passarello, MD
Infectious Diarrhea

Scott Schmidt, MD
Anuj Parikh, MD
*Peritonitis/Perforated
Viscous/Intra-Abdominal
Abscess*

Kristine Schultz, MD
Kelly Harrison, PA-C
*Varicella/ Chicken Pox/
Zoster/Shingles*

Kristine Schultz, MD
John Jesus, MD
Balanitis

Stephen Senichka, MD
Angelo Grillo, MD
Bartholin's Cyst/Abscess

Sarah Shafer, MD
George Zlupko, MD
*Conjunctivitis
Peritoneal Dialysis-
Related Peritonitis*

Erum Siddiqui, MD
Kristina Stransky, MD
*Rocky Mountain
Spotted Fever*

Jason Stankiewicz, MD
Paul Sierzenski, MD
Scabies/Mites

Justin Stowens, MD
Matthew Barrett, DO
Pneumonia, Adult

Justin Stowens, MD
Lori Felker, PA-C
Mastitis

Nicholas Surra, MD
Paul Anderson, MD
Impetigo

Nicholas Surra, MD
Eli Zeserson, MD
*Pseudomembranous
Colitis*

Orel Swenson, MD
Robert Rosenbaum, MD
Endometritis

Andrew Tee, MD
Arayel Osborne, MD
Bronchitis

Emilio Volz, MD
Stephen Koczirka, MD
Influenza

Emilio Volz, MD
Theresa Nguyen, MD
Bell's Palsy

Danielle Whitley, MD
Ross Megargel, DO
Spinal Epidural Abscess

Danielle Whitley, MD
Tim Shiuh, MD
Epididymitis/Orchitis

Michael Wiedner, MD
William Paynter, PA-C
*Common Pediatric
Antibiotic Dosing*

Michael Wiedner, MD
Michelle Shaw, PA-C
Sinusitis

Mary-Stewart Willsie, DO
Brian Burgess, MD
Cellulitis/Erysipelas

Mary-Stewart Willsie, DO
Joseph Zaweski, PA-C
*Parapharyngeal
Abscess (Peritonsillar
and Retropharyngeal)*

Peer Review
Casey M. Clements, M.D., Ph.D.
Assistant Professor of Emergency Medicine
Department of Emergency Medicine
Mayo Clinic
Rochester, MN

TABLE OF CONTENTS

TABLE OF CONTENTS

SEPTIC BURSITIS

Common organisms: *S. aureus, Streptococcus spp.,* polymicrobial

Mild Inflammation: Outpatient Treatment (if not diabetic or immunocompromised, duration 2–3 weeks)
- TMP/SMX 1–2 DS tabs (5 mg TMP/kg) PO two times daily
- Clindamycin 600 mg (10 mg/kg) PO three times daily

Severe Inflammation: Inpatient Treatment
- Clindamycin 600 mg (10 mg/kg) IV three times daily
- Vancomycin 15–20 mg/kg IV two times daily (15 mg/kg IV four times daily)
- Linezolid 600 mg IV two times daily (10 mg/kg IV three times daily)

PEARLS
- Low WBC count and negative gram stain do not rule out infection.
- Olecranon and prepatellar bursae prone to infection from local trauma.

DISCITIS/VERTEBRAL OSTEOMYELITIS

Common organisms: *S. aureus, Streptococcus spp., Pseudomonas spp., E. coli, M. tuberculosis*
- Vancomycin 15–20 mg/kg IV two times daily **PLUS**
  - Ceftriaxone 2 g IV once daily (no *Pseudomonas* coverage) **OR**
  - Ceftazidime 2 g IV three times daily **OR**
  - Cefepime 2 g IV three times daily **OR**
  - Ciprofloxacin 400 mg IV three times daily

PEARLS
- Consider withholding empiric antimicrobial therapy until microbiologic diagnosis is confirmed in a stable patient without neurologic deficits.
- Risk factors include IVDA, endocarditis, prior spinal surgery, diabetes, corticosteroid therapy.
- ESR elevated >80% of cases; local tenderness to gentle spinal percussion is the most reliable clinical sign.
- Culture of blood, bone, and/or disc is essential for identification of causative agent.
- X-ray often normal, but may show narrowing of disc space and irregularity of adjacent vertebral end-plates.
- MRI is the diagnostic imaging modality of choice.

OPEN FRACTURES

Common organisms: *S. aureus,* coagulase-negative staphylococci, polymicrobial

Open Fracture
- Type I or II injury
  - Cefazolin 2 g (30 mg/kg) IV three times daily
  - Vancomycin 15–20 mg/kg IV two times daily (15 mg/kg IV four times daily)
  - Ciprofloxacin 400 mg IV two times daily
- Type III injury
  - Choose one from above and **ADD** gentamicin 5–7 mg/kg IV once daily (2.5 mg/kg IV three times daily)
- If concern for *Clostridia* due to farm injury, soil contamination, or vascular injury
  - Piperacillin/tazobactam 4.5 g (80 mg/kg) IV three times daily as **monotherapy**

PEARLS
- Administer copious irrigation and antibiotics as soon as possible post-injury.
- Address tetanus immunization status.
- Type I – open fracture with <1 cm clean laceration and minimal soft tissue damage.
- Type II – open fracture with >1 cm clean laceration without extensive soft tissue injury, flaps, or avulsion.
- Type III – open fracture with extensive soft tissue damage including muscle, skin, and neurovascular structures; a traumatic amputation, arterial injury that requires repair, or heavily contaminated/farm injury.

OSTEOMYELITIS

Adult: Empiric Regimen (including sickle cell disease and IV drug users)

Common organisms: *S. aureus,* coagulase-negative staphylococci, and aerobic gram-negative bacilli

- Vancomycin 15–20 mg/kg IV two times daily *OR* linezolid 600 mg IV two times daily *OR* daptomycin 6 mg/kg IV
  PLUS
  - Ceftriaxone 2 g IV once daily *OR*
  - Ciprofloxacin 400 mg IV three times daily *OR*
  - Cefepime 2 g IV two-three times daily

Adult: Puncture Wound

Common organisms: *P. aeruginosa*

- Ciprofloxacin 400 mg IV three times daily or 750 mg PO two times daily
- Cefepime 2 g IV two-three times daily
- Ceftazidime 2 g IV two times daily

Note: Consider MRSA coverage.

Pediatric: Neonates to 3 Months

Common organisms: *S. aureus,* gram-negative rods, *group B streptococcus*

- Cefotaxime 50 mg/kg IV three times daily ***PLUS***
  - Nafcillin/oxacillin 25–50 mg/kg IV two-three times daily *OR*
  - Vancomycin 15 mg/kg IV three-four times daily (if prolonged NICU stay)

Pediatric: Older Infants and Children

Common organisms: *S. aureus, group A streptococcus*

- Vancomycin 15 mg/kg IV four times daily
- Nafcillin/oxacillin 25–50 mg/kg IV four times daily
- Clindamycin 10 mg/kg IV/PO four times daily

Pediatric: Sickle Cell Disease (or concern not vaccinated against Hib)

Common organisms: *Salmonella, S. aureus*

- Ceftriaxone 50 mg/kg IV once daily *OR* cefotaxime 50 mg/kg IV three times daily
  PLUS
  — Vancomycin 15 mg/kg IV four times daily *OR*
  — Clindamycin 10 mg/kg IV/PO four times daily *OR*

Pediatric: Puncture Wound

Common organisms: *P. aeruginosa* and/or *S. aureus*

- Ceftazidime 50 mg/kg IV three times daily
- Cefepime 50 mg/kg IV three times daily

Note: Consider MRSA coverage.

PEARLS

- Hardware involvement: Consider *ADDING* rifampin 600 mg IV daily after discussing with infectious disease consultant.
- Ability to probe to bone on exam confirms diagnosis, until proven otherwise.
- A normal x-ray does not exclude diagnosis. X-ray findings such as cortical erosion, periosteal thickening, mixed lucency, and sclerosis lag at least 2 weeks behind clinical infection.
- Bone biopsy is the gold standard; soft-tissue wound cultures do not reliably correlate with actual organism causing the osteomyelitis.
- MRI for diabetic infections or suspected vertebral osteomyelitis (CT if MRI unavailable). Nuclear studies (bone scan, gallium scan, white blood cell scan) for patients with metal hardware.

SEPTIC ARTHRITIS

Adult: Non-Gonococcal

Common organisms: *S. aureus, Streptococcus spp., Pseudomonas spp., Enterococcus, B. burgdorferi*

- Vancomycin 15–20 mg/kg IV two times daily **PLUS**
  — Ceftriaxone 2 g IV once daily *OR*
  — Cefepime 2 g IV three times daily *OR*
  — Ceftazidime 2 g IV three times daily *OR*
  — Ciprofloxacin 400 mg IV three times daily

14

Adult: Gonococcal
- Ceftriaxone 1 g IV once daily

Sickle Cell

Common organisms: *Salmonella spp, Staphylococcus spp*
- Vancomycin 15–20 mg/kg IV two times daily **PLUS**
  — Ciprofloxacin 400 mg IV three times daily **OR**
  — Imipenem 500 mg IV four times daily

Pediatric

Common organisms: *S. aureus, Streptococcus spp., N. gonorrhea, Enterobacter spp.*, gram-negative species
- Vancomycin 15 mg/kg IV four times daily **PLUS**
  — Ceftriaxone 100 mg/kg IV daily (max 2 g) **OR**
  — Cefotaxime 50 mg/kg IV four times daily

PEARLS
- Hardware involvement: Consider **ADDING** rifampin 600 mg IV once daily after discussing with infectious diseases consultant.
- Joint aspirate WBC >50,000 and PMN predominance is associated with septic arthritis, although up to 1/3 may have less.
- Send synovial fluid for gram stain, culture, cell count, and crystal analysis. Sending aspirated fluid to the lab in blood culture bottles may increase culture yield.
- Consider gonococcal infections in polyarticular arthritis.
- Culture blood, urethra, cervix, urine, and joint fluid if gonorrhea suspected. Additional cultures of throat and anus may be required.
- All patients treated for a gonococcal infection should also receive a 7-day course of doxycycline or 1 gram azithromycin to cover the possibility of a concurrent infection with *Chlamydia trachomatis*.

INFECTIOUS TENOSYNOVITIS

Healthy, *without* Bite Wound

Common organisms: *S. aureus, Streptococcus spp.*
- Vancomycin 15–20 mg/kg IV two times daily **PLUS**
  — Ceftriaxone 1 g IV daily **OR**
  — Levofloxacin 750 mg IV daily

Gonococcal

- Ceftriaxone 1 g IV once daily

Immunocompromised or Bite Wound, ADULT

Common organisms: *S. aureus, Streptococcus spp., Fusobacterium, Bacteroides spp., Pasteurella multocida (cat), Eikenella corrodens (human), Capnocytophaga canimorsus (dog)*

- Ampicillin/sulbactam 3 g IV four times daily
- Piperacillin/tazobactam 4.5 g IV three times daily
- Ceftriaxone 1 g IV daily **AND** metronidazole 500 mg IV three times daily
- Levofloxacin 750 mg IV daily **AND** metronidazole 500 mg IV three times daily
- Levofloxacin 750 mg IV daily **AND** clindamycin 600 mg IV three times daily
- If MRSA suspected, **ADD** vancomycin 15–20 mg/kg IV two times daily

Immunocompromised or Bite Wound, PEDIATRIC

Common organisms: as above

- Ampicillin/sulbactam 50 mg/kg IV four times daily
- Ceftriaxone 100 mg/kg IV once daily **AND** metronidazole 7.5 mg/kg IV four times daily
- Clindamycin 10 mg/kg IV three times daily **AND** TMP/SMX 5 mg/kg IV two times daily
- If MRSA suspected, **ADD** vancomycin 15 mg/kg IV four times daily

PEARLS

- Immediate surgical consult is required.
- Remember tetanus prophylaxis.
- Kanavel's four cardinal signs: "sausage digit," held in slight flexion, tenderness along flexor tendon sheath, and pain with passive extension.
- For water-related injuries, consider mycobacteria (clarithromycin 500 mg PO two times daily **AND** either ethambutol 15 mg/kg PO once daily **OR** rifampin 600 mg PO once daily) and *Pseudomonas* (levofloxacin 750 mg PO once daily).
- Suspect gonorrhea if rash, polyarthralgias, and fever are present.
  - Vaginal or penile discharge is usually absent.
  - Consider culturing urethra, cervix, anus, throat, blood, and joint fluid prior to treatment.
  - Treat for possible concurrent *Chlamydia trachomatis* infection.

ENDOCARDITIS

Native Valve

Common organisms: *Viridans group streptococci, S. aureus, Streptococcus spp., Enterococcus spp.*

- Oxacillin/nafcillin 2 g IV six times daily *AND* gentamicin 1 mg/kg IV three times daily *AND* ampicillin 2 g IV six times daily
- Vancomycin 15–20 mg/kg IV two times daily *AND* gentamicin 1 mg/kg IV three times daily
- Daptomycin 6 mg/kg IV once daily

Prosthetic Valve

Common organisms:
 <2 mos post-op: Coagulase-negative staphylococci, *S. aureus*
 >2 mos post-op: Coagulase-negative staphylococci, *viridans group streptococci, S. aureus, Enterococcus spp.*

- Vancomycin 15–20 mg/kg IV two times daily *AND* rifampin 300 mg PO/IV three times daily *AND* gentamicin 1 mg/kg IV three times daily

IV Drug Use

Common organism: *S. aureus*

- Vancomycin 15–20 mg/kg IV two times daily
- Daptomycin 6 mg/kg IV once daily

PEARLS

- Three sets of blood cultures is standard practice for diagnosis. These cultures should be drawn 20 minutes apart and BEFORE giving antibiotics, provided that the patient is stable (i.e., not in heart failure).
- Consider a loading dose of vancomycin (25–30 mg/kg) for seriously ill patients.
- A transesophageal echocardiogram may be necessary to assess for vegetation and the degree of heart failure.
- Implanted devices should not have the pocket sampled; definitive treatment requires exploration.

BELL'S PALSY

Common organisms: *Herpes simplex virus (HSV), herpes zoster,*
B. burgdorferi (Lyme)

PEARLS

- Send Lyme titer in endemic areas; use clinical judgment to treat.
- Ensure proper eye protection with artificial tears to prevent corneal ulceration during recovery.
- 85% of patients will have complete recovery in 3–6 months. 85% of patients see some recovery in 3 weeks.
- Imaging is not necessary unless there are recurrent or additional neurologic findings or suspected trauma.
- Literature supports an improved rate of recovery if steroids are used within 72 hours of onset (for patients aged 16 and over).
  — Prednisolone 60 mg PO daily for 5 days followed by a taper
  — Prednisolone 25 mg PO two times daily for 10 days
- Antivirals have not been shown to provide any additional recovery benefit — only treat with antivirals if high suspicion for HSV.
- If HSV highly suspected, in addition to steroids, give:
  — Acyclovir 400 mg PO five times daily (20 mg/kg PO four times daily, max dose 1000 mg/day) for 10 days
  — Valacyclovir 1 g PO three times daily for 7–10 days

ENCEPHALITIS

Most common pathogens are HSV, VZV, and CMV. Other causes include Rickettsial and Ehrlichial infections, arboviruses (i.e., West Nile), EBV, CMV, HHV6 and toxoplasmosis.

Herpes Simplex/Varicella Zoster Viruses

- Acyclovir 10 mg/kg (20 mg/kg) IV three times daily

Cytomegalovirus

- Ganciclovir 5 mg/kg IV two times daily *AND* foscarnet 90 mg/kg IV two times daily

PEARLS

- Start acyclovir empirically as it has been shown to decrease morbidity in HSV encephalitis.
- Acyclovir dosing is based on *ideal* body weight, not *actual* body weight

- Most viral encephalitides are not treatable beyond supportive care with the exception of HSV/VZV.
- In addition to routine CSF studies, obtain cultures for PCR for HSV, CMV, and VZV.
- For immunocompromised patients, consider treatment for Toxoplasmosis (page 83).

INTRACRANIAL ABSCESS

Common organisms: *Streptococcus spp., Bacteroides spp., Enterobacteriaceae, S. aureus, Toxoplasma*
- Vancomycin 15–20 mg/kg IV two times daily (10 mg/kg IV four times daily) **AND**
- Ceftriaxone 2 g (50 mg/kg) IV two times daily **PLUS**
  - Metronidazole 500 mg (7.5 mg/kg) IV four times daily **OR**
  - Clindamycin 600–900 mg IV three times daily (10 mg/kg IV four times daily)
- If PCN allergic: replace ceftriaxone with aztreonam 2 g (30 mg/kg) IV four times daily

PEARLS
- MRI with and without gadolinium is the test of choice; if MRI is unavailable, CT with contrast is recommended.
- Consider coverage for fungal, toxoplasmosis, or tuberculous infections in immunocompromised patients.
- Glucocorticoid use is controversial, but can be used when substantial mass effect can be demonstrated on imaging and the mental status is significantly depressed.

SPINAL EPIDURAL ABSCESS

Common organisms: *S. aureus, coagulase-negative staphylococci, Streptococcus spp., anaerobes, gram-negative bacilli*
- Vancomycin 15–20 mg/kg IV two times daily (10 mg/kg IV four times daily) **AND** Ceftriaxone 2 g (50 mg/kg) IV two times daily **PLUS**
  - Metronidazole 500 mg (7.5 mg/kg) IV four times daily **OR**
  - Clindamycin 600–900 mg IV three times daily (10 mg/kg IV four times daily)

- If pseudomonas suspected, replace ceftriaxone with
  - Cefepime 2 g (50 mg/kg) IV three times daily

PEARLS

- Immediate neurosurgical intervention should not be delayed, even in patients who are neurologically intact.
- MRI is the diagnostic test of choice.
- ESR has been shown to be a sensitive screening tool.
- Classic triad of back pain, fever, and neurologic deficit only occurs in 13%.

MENINGITIS

Neonate to 1 Month

Common organisms: *Group B streptococcus (GBS), E. coli, Listeria spp., Klebsiella spp.*

- Ampicillin 50 mg/kg IV four times daily (three times daily <1wk old) *PLUS*
  - Cefotaxime 50 mg/kg IV four times daily (three times daily <1 wk old) **OR**
  - Gentamicin 2.5 mg/kg IV three times daily (two times daily <1 wk old)
- If MRSA suspected, *ADD* vancomycin 10 mg/kg IV four times daily (three times daily <1 wk old)
- Consider coverage for herpes meningoencephalitis with acyclovir 20 mg/kg IV three times daily

1 Month to Adult

Common organisms: *S. pneumoniae, N. meningitidis* (*GBS, E. coli,* and *H. influenzae* for 1 to 23 months old)

- Vancomycin 15–20 mg/kg IV two times daily (15 mg/kg IV four times daily) *PLUS*
- Ceftriaxone 2 g (50 mg/kg) IV two times daily
  - Consider coverage for herpes meningoencephalitis with acyclovir 10 mg/kg (20 mg/kg) IV three times daily
  - If *Listeria* suspected (>50 years old) or immunocompromised, *ADD* ampicillin 2 g IV six times daily (75 mg/kg IV four times daily)
  - If penicillin allergic: replace ceftriaxone with chloramphenicol 1.5 g (25 mg/kg) IV four times daily *AND* if *Listeria* suspected, *ADD* TMP/SMX 5 mg/kg IV four times daily

Post-neurosurgery, Penetrating Head Trauma, CSF Shunt

Common organisms: Gram-negative rods, *S. aureus, propionibacterium (CSF shunt)*

- Vancomycin 15–20 mg/kg IV two times daily (15 mg/kg IV four times daily) *PLUS*
  - Cefepime 2 g (50 mg/kg) IV three times daily *OR*
  - Ceftazidime 2 g (50 mg/kg) IV three times daily *OR*
  - Meropenem 2 g (40 mg/kg) IV three times daily

Cryptococcal Meningitis

- Amphotericin B deoxycholate 0.7–1 mg/kg IV daily *AND* flucytosine 25 mg/kg PO four times daily
- Amphotericin B (liposomal) 4 mg/kg IV daily *AND* flucytosine 25 mg/kg PO four times daily
- Amphotericin B (lipid complex) 5 mg/kg IV daily *AND* flucytosine 25 mg/kg PO four times daily

Suspected Tuberculous Meningitis

- Isoniazid 300 mg (10–15 mg/kg) PO once daily *AND* rifampin 600 mg (10–20 mg/kg) PO/IV once daily *AND* pyrazinamide 2 g (15–30 mg/kg) PO once daily *AND* ethambutol 1600 mg (15–20 mg/kg) PO once daily

Prophylaxis for Neisseria Meningitidis (not recommended for other organisms)

For all household contacts; child care/nursery school contact or DIRECT exposure to patient's body fluids occurring within 7 days prior to patient presentation.

- Ceftriaxone 250 mg IM once (≤15 years old, 125 mg IM)
- Ciprofloxacin 500 mg PO once
- Rifampin 600 mg (<1 month old, 5 mg/kg; ≥1 month old, 10 mg/kg) PO two times daily for 2 days

PEARLS

- Some experts advocate loading vancomycin (25–30 mg/kg).
- Acyclovir dosing is based on *ideal* body weight, not *actual* body weight.
- Do not delay antibiotic therapy for LP or imaging.
- CT should be done prior to lumbar puncture only if one or more of the following exist:
  - Immunocompromised states, history of CNS disease: Mass lesion, stroke, or focal infection, new onset seizure, papilledema, abnormal level of consciousness, focal neurological deficit
- For highly suspected pneumoccal meningitis, consider dexamethasone (0.15 mg/kg IV four times daily for two to four days) BEFORE the first dose of antibiotics.

ACUTE NECROTIZING ULCERATIVE GINGIVITIS (ANUG)

Common organisms: *Fusobacterium, Prevotella, Tannerella,* other oral spirochetes

- Amoxicillin 500 mg PO three times daily **AND** metronidazole 500 mg PO three times daily
- Amoxicillin-clavulanate 875 mg PO two times daily
- Clindamycin 450 mg PO three times daily **OR** 600 mg IV three times daily
- Ampicillin/sulbactam 3 g IV four times daily
- If HIV-positive, consider
  - Nystatin rinses 5 ml four times daily for 7–14 days
  - Fluconazole 200 mg PO daily for 7–14 days

PEARLS

- Outpatient regimen is for 10 days.
- Diagnostic triad includes pain, ulcerated interdental papillae, and gingival bleeding.
- Often sudden onset and may include gingival edema, gray pseudomembranes over ulcerations, and halitosis.
- May progress to Vincent's angina (tonsillar, pharyngeal involvement): searing pharyngeal pain, fever, and regional lymphadenopathy.

DENTAL ABSCESS

Common organisms: Polymicrobial oral flora

- Penicillin VK 500 mg PO four times daily for 7 days
- Amoxicillin/clavulanate 875 mg PO two times daily for 7 days
- Clindamycin 450 mg PO three times daily for 10 days or 600–900 mg IV three times daily
- Ampicillin/sulbactam 3 g IV four times daily

PEARLS

- Three days of therapy can be considered with appropriate follow-up with source control.
- Surgical drainage is recommended.

EPIGLOTTITIS

Common organisms: Group A Streptococcus, *H. parainfluenzae, S. pneumoniae, S. aureus, H. influenzae*
- Ceftriaxone 2 g (50 mg/kg) IV once daily
- Ampicillin/sulbactam 3 g (50 mg/kg) IV four times daily
- Levofloxacin 750 mg IV once daily

Severe Infection or Immunocompromised Patient

Common organisms: As above *PLUS C. albicans, Pseudomonas spp., M. tuberculosis, MRSA*
- Cefepime 2 g (50 mg/kg) IV three times daily *AND* vancomycin 15–20 mg/kg IV two times daily (15 mg/kg IV four times daily)
- Consider adding antifungal agent in consultation with infectious disease.

PEARLS
- Patients with appropriate clinical picture: dyspnea, stridor, and tripod positioning warrant early intubation in a controlled setting (patient may require surgical airway).
- All non-intubated patients warrant close monitoring of airway. ICU admission is recommended.
- Use of steroids and racemic epinephrine is controversial.
- Consider prophylaxis for close contacts of suspected *H. influenzae* with rifampin 20 mg/kg PO (600 mg max) once daily for 4 days (especially important in children < age 4, children without primary vaccination, or immunocompromised contacts).

LUDWIG'S ANGINA

Common organisms: *Polymicrobial oral flora*

Immunocompetent
- Clindamycin 600 mg IV three times daily (10 mg/kg IV four times daily)
- Ampicillin/sulbactam 3 g (50 mg/kg) IV four times daily
- Penicillin G 4 million units (50,000 units) IV four times daily *AND* metronidazole 500 mg IV three times daily (7.5 mg/kg four times daily)

Immunocompromised

- Piperacillin/tazobactam 4.5 g (80 mg/kg) IV three times daily
- Imipenem/cilastatin 500 mg (20 mg/kg) IV four times daily
- Cefepime 2 g (50 mg/kg) IV two times daily *AND* metronidazole 500 mg IV three times daily (7.5 mg/kg four times daily)

PEARLS

- May consider adding vancomycin 15–20 mg/kg IV two times daily for MRSA coverage.
- Clinical findings: "hot potato" voice, dysphagia, drooling, stridor, trismus, tongue elevation, edema of the floor of mouth, and a high fever.
- One-third require fiberoptic intubation or tracheostomy.
- CT clarifies extent of infection.
- Obtain early ENT or surgical involvement.

MASTOIDITIS

Common organisms: *S. pneumoniae, S. pyogenes, S. aureus, H. influenzae*

- Vancomycin 15–20 mg/kg IV two times daily (15 mg/kg IV four times daily) *PLUS*
  - Ceftriaxone 1 g (50 mg/kg) IV once daily *OR*
  - Ampicillin/sulbactam 3 g (50 mg/kg) IV four times daily
- Clindamycin 600 mg IV three times daily (10 mg/kg IV four times daily)

PEARLS

- Presents as acute otitis media *PLUS* postauricular edema, erythema, tenderness, displacement of the auricle.
- Consider CT or MRI of temporal bones and intracranial cavity to exclude osteomyelitis or abscess.
- Patients with mild mastoiditis may be treated as outpatients. See *Otitis Media chapter* for treatment recommendations.
- Chronic mastoiditis requires ENT consultation for management recommendations.

OTITIS EXTERNA

Acute Otitis Externa (swimmer's ear)

Common organisms: *Pseudomonas aeruginosa, Staphylococcus spp., Peptostreptococcus spp., Bacteroides spp.* (treatment duration: 7 days)

- Polymyxin B/neomycin/hydrocortisone 5 drops four times daily (also treatment of choice for chronic otitis externa)
- Ofloxacin 0.3% otic solution 10 drops once daily
- Ciprofloxacin/hydrocortisone 3 drops two times daily
- Ciprofloxacin 500 mg PO two times daily for 7–10 days (for severe acute otitis externa or immunocompromised patient)

PEARLS

- Consider cerumen removal to expedite resolution.
- Avoid aminoglycosides in patients with tympanostomy tubes or suspected TM rupture.
- Acidifying the ear canal with acetic acid may help inhibit bacterial and fungal growth.
- Infuse wick with antibiotic for 48 hours if external ear canal is edematous with obstruction.
- Consider topical analgesic drops for comfort.

Malignant Otitis Externa

Common organisms: *Pseudomonas aeruginosa*

- Ciprofloxacin 400 mg IV three times daily **OR** 750 mg PO two times daily (15 mg/kg IV/PO two times daily)
- Piperacillin/tazobactam 4.5 g (100 mg/kg) IV four times daily
- Cefepime 2 g (50 mg/kg) IV three times daily
- Imipenem/cilastatin 500 mg (25 mg/kg) IV four times daily

PEARLS

- Consider oral ciprofloxacin for treatment of patients with early disease.
- Consider antifungals in the appropriate setting: diabetics, immunocompromised (AIDS, chemotherapy).
- Consider CT or MRI scan to determine extent of disease.
- Consider admission for IV antibiotics and possible surgical debridement.

OTITIS MEDIA

Common organisms: *S. pneumoniae, H. influenzae, M. catarrhalis,
S. pyogenes, S. aureus, respiratory viruses*

No Antibiotics in Prior Month (treatment duration: 7–10 days)
- Amoxicillin 45 mg/kg PO two times daily

Antibiotics in Prior Month (treatment duration: 7–10 days)
- Amoxicillin/clavulanate 45 mg/kg PO two times daily
- Cefdinir 14 mg/kg PO once daily
- Cefpodoxime 5 mg/kg PO two times daily
- Cefuroxime 15 mg/kg PO two times daily

Treatment Failure (treatment duration: 7–10 days)
- Amoxicillin/clavulanate 45 mg/kg PO two times daily
- Ceftriaxone 50 mg/kg IM (max 1000mg) once daily for 3 days

Severe Penicillin Allergy
- Clindamycin 10 mg/kg PO three times daily (does not cover *H. influenzae* or *M. catarrhalis*)
- Azithromycin 10 mg/kg PO once daily for day 1, *THEN* 5 mg/kg PO once daily for days 2 through 5

PEARLS

- Consider symptomatic treatment (NSAIDS, topical benzocaine/antipyrine) with 48- to 72-hour follow up in non-severe, unilateral AOM in children >6 months.
- Indications for antibiotics include otorrhea, severe symptoms (toxic appearance, otalgia >48 hours, T >39°C), or poor follow up.
- Amoxicillin/clavulanate recommended for otitis-conjunctivitis syndrome.
- Definition of treatment failure: no change in ear pain, fever, bulging TM, otorrhea after three days treatment.
- Can consider cephalosporins despite mild PCN reactions (non-Type I).
- Persistent middle ear effusion is common after the resolution of acute symptoms.

PAROTITIS

Common organisms: *S. aureus,* oral flora, mumps virus, enteroviruses, influenza virus

- Amoxicillin/clavulanate 875 mg (45 mg/kg) PO two times daily
- Cephalexin 500 mg (12.5 mg/kg) PO four times daily
- Clindamycin 450 mg (10 mg/kg) PO three times daily

Intravenous Treatment

- Vancomycin 15–20 mg/kg IV two times daily (15 mg/kg IV four times daily) **OR** linezolid 600 mg IV two times daily **PLUS**
  - Metronidazole 500 mg IV three times daily
  - Clindamycin 600 mg IV three times daily
  - Ampicillin/sulbactam 3 g IV four times daily

PEARLS

- Treatment duration is 10–14 days for uncomplicated cases.
- Consider broad gram-negative coverage if diabetic or immunocompromised.
- Highest risk for bacterial infection is over 60 y/o, chronically ill, or diabetic.
- Dehydration is a risk factor for bacterial parotitis.
- Consider establishing duct patency with massage or stimulation of salivary glands with sialogogues (lemon drops or orange juice).

PARAPHARYNGEAL ABSCESS (PERITONSILLAR AND RETROPHARYNGEAL)

Common organisms: *Streptococcus spp.,* anaerobes, *Eikenella corrodens, H. influenzae, S. aureus*

Outpatient

- Amoxicillin/clavulanate 875 mg PO (45 mg/kg) two times daily
- Clindamycin 450 mg (10 mg/kg) PO three times daily

Inpatient

- Ampicillin/sulbactam 3 g (50 mg/kg) IV four times daily
- Clindamycin 600 mg IV three times daily (10 mg/kg IV four times daily)

- Penicillin G 4 million units (50,000 units/kg) IV four times daily **AND** metronidazole 500 mg IV three times daily (7.5 mg/kg IV four times daily)

PEARLS

- Imaging options: CT neck with IV contrast, intra-oral ultrasound or lateral neck radiograph.
- Incision and drainage is often necessary.
- Consider steroids for symptomatic relief (dexamethasone 0.6 mg/kg **OR** 10 mg maximum).

PERTUSSIS

Common organism: *Bordetella spp.*

<1 month, Active Disease/Post-Exposure Prophylaxis
- Azithromycin 10 mg/kg PO once daily for 5 days (max 500 mg/day)

>1 month, Active Disease/Post-Exposure Prophylaxis
- Azithromycin 10 mg/kg (max 500 mg/day) PO once daily for 5 days (1–5 months)
- Azithromycin 10 mg/kg (max 500 mg) PO once daily for day 1, **THEN** 5 mg/kg (max 250 mg/day) PO once daily for days 2 through 5 (>6 months)
- TMP/SMX 4 mg/kg PO two times daily for 14 days (>2 months)

Adult, Active Disease/Post-Exposure Prophylaxis
- Azithromycin 500 mg PO once daily for day 1, **THEN** 250 mg PO once daily for days 2 through 5
- TMP/SMX (DS) 1 tablet PO two times daily for 14 days

PEARLS

- Classically, a pediatric illness; however, immunity wanes 10 years after immunization. Single dose of Tdap recommended for individuals >10 years old.
- Extremely contagious (via respiratory droplet) in non-immunized children and adults (>80% of susceptible individuals exposed will develop the illness). Average incubation period is 7–10 days. Most infectious in catarrhal stage or the first 3 weeks of cough symptoms.
- Consider in any patient with prolonged cough, coughing paroxysms, whoops, or post-tussive emesis.

- Pertussis is a clinical diagnosis, but can be confirmed through nasopharyngeal culture (gold standard) or PCR.
- Complications (most common in unvaccinated youth) include hypoxia, apnea, pneumonia, seizures, encephalopathy, and malnutrition.
- Post-exposure prophylaxis recommended for close contacts, especially infants and pregnant women.

SINUSITIS (ACUTE)

Common organisms: *Viral, S. pneumoniae, H. influenza, M. catarrhalis*
Note: 90–98% of cases are viral. NSAIDS, antipyretics, intra-nasal saline irrigation and intranasal corticosteroids may provide symptomatic relief. Oral or intranasal decongestants should be avoided in suspected bacterial sinusitis.

Mild to Moderate Disease (treatment duration: 5–7 days)
- Amoxicillin/clavulanate 875 mg PO two times daily
- Doxycycline 100 mg PO two times daily

Pediatric Dosing (treatment duration: 10–14 days)
- Amoxicillin/clavulanate 45 mg/kg PO two times daily
- Levofloxacin 10 mg/kg PO one to two times daily (>6 months old)

Risk for Resistance or Antibiotic Failure (outpatient)
- Amoxicillin/clavulanate 2000 mg (90 mg/kg) PO two times daily for 10–14 days
- Levofloxacin 500 mg PO once daily for 5 days (10 mg/kg one to two times daily for 10–14 days)
- Moxifloxacin 400 mg PO once daily for 10 days

Severe Disease (inpatient)
- Ampicillin/sulbactam 3g (50 mg/kg) IV four times daily
- Levofloxacin 500 mg IV once daily (10 mg/kg one to two times daily)
- Moxifloxacin 400 mg IV once daily
- Ceftriaxone 1g IV one to two times daily (50 mg/kg two times daily)

PEARLS
- Indications for antibiotics: No symptom improvement after 10 days; onset with high fever ≥39°C and purulent nasal discharge, or facial pain for at least 3–4 days; worsening symptoms following viral URI that lasted 5–6 days and was initially improving.
- Antibiotic failure: worsening symptoms or no improvement after 3–5 days of initial treatment.

- Risk for resistance: severe infection, attendance at daycare, age <2 or >65 years, recent hospitalization, antibiotic use within past month, or if immunocompromised.
- Severe disease: evidence of systemic toxicity, fever ≥39°C, and threat of suppurative complications.
- For severe, complicated, or refractory disease: consider CT imaging of sinuses and inpatient admission with IV vancomycin for MRSA or highly resistant *S. pneumoniae* coverage; obtaining cultures by direct sinus aspiration; consult with ENT and ID for possible antifungal therapy.

THRUSH

Common organism: *Candida spp.*

Adult Dosing
Mild Disease
- Clotrimazole troches 10 mg PO five times daily for 14 days (dissolve over 20 minutes)
- Nystatin oral suspension (100,000 units/ml) 5 ml PO four times daily for 14 days (swish and swallow over 20 minutes)

Moderate to Severe Disease
- Fluconazole 200 mg PO once, *THEN* 100 mg PO once daily for 13 days

Refractory Disease
- Itraconazole oral solution 200 mg PO once daily without food for 14 days
- Posaconazole suspension 400 mg PO two times daily for 3 days, *THEN* 400 mg PO daily for up to 28 days
- Voriconazole 200 mg PO two times daily for 14 days

Pediatric Dosing
- Clotrimazole troches (if >3 years old) 10 mg PO five times daily for 14 days (dissolve over 20 minutes)
- Nystatin oral suspension (100,000 units/ml); 14 days for all groups
  - Premature/low birth-weight infants: 0.5 ml to each side of mouth four times daily
  - Infants: 1 ml to each side of mouth four times daily
  - Children: 5 ml PO four times daily (swish and swallow)
- Fluconazole (if >14 days old) 6 mg/kg PO once, *THEN* 3 mg/kg PO once daily for 13 (100 mg/day max)

PEARLS

- Predisposing factors include dentures, use of steroid inhaler, HIV, leukemia, malnutrition, radiation or chemotherapy treatment, and chronic immunosuppressive therapy.
- Thrush usually resolves within 3–4 days of treatment. Discontinue treatment 2 days after lesions disappear.
- Apply the nystatin directly on the lesions with a cotton swab or finger.
- Treat dentures as well as oral cavity to prevent recurrences (brush dentures and soak in chlorhexidine gluconate solution nightly).
- If breastfeeding, mothers must also treat their nipples after each feeding.
- If bottle feeding, sterilize the nipples prior to feeding.

TONSILLITIS/PHARYNGITIS

Common organisms: *Viruses (mononucleosis, adenovirus, coxsackievirus, HIV, HSV), Group A beta-hemolytic Streptococcus (GABHS), N. gonorrhea, C. diphtheriae*

Adult (treatment duration: 10 days unless otherwise noted)
- Benzathine penicillin G 1.2 million units IM once
- Penicillin VK 500 mg PO two times daily
- Amoxicillin 1000 mg PO once daily
- Cephalexin 500 mg PO two times daily
- Azithromycin 500 mg PO once daily for 5 days
- Clindamycin 300 mg PO three times daily

Pediatric (treatment duration: 10 days unless otherwise noted)
- Benzathine penicillin G <27 kg 600,000 units IM once, ≥27 kg 1.2 million units IM once
- Penicillin VK <27 kg 25 0mg PO twice or three times daily, ≥27 kg 500 mg PO twice daily
- Amoxicillin 25 mg/kg PO two times daily (max = 500 mg/dose) **OR** 50 mg/kg PO once daily (max = 1000 mg)
- Cephalexin 20 mg/kg PO two times daily (max = 500 mg/dose)
- Cefadroxil 30 mg/kg PO once daily (max = 1 g)
- Azithromycin 12 mg/kg PO once daily for 5 days (max = 500 mg)
- Clindamycin 7 mg/kg PO three times daily (max = 300 mg/dose)

PEARLS

- GABHS is responsible for 5–15% of sore throat visits in adults, and 20–30% in children.
- Modified Centor Criteria are often used to decrease unnecessary antibiotic use in pharyngitis: 1) tonsillar exudate; 2) fever or history of fever >38 C; 3) tender anterior cervical lymphadenopathy; 4) absence of cough; and 5) age >3 and <15 (age ≥45 = subtract 1 point)
  - 0–2 points: antibiotic treatment generally not indicated
  - 3–5 points: consider antibiotic treatment
  - 1–3 points: consider rapid antigen detection testing or throat culture if feasible
- Symptomatic treatment with warmed fluids, topical anesthetics, gargles, steroids (dexamethasone 0.6 mg/kg or 10 mg max), and acetaminophen or ibuprofen.
- Monospot tests and peripheral blood smears for suspected mononucleosis if symptoms present >1 week; supportive treatment with steroids, hydration, supplemental oxygen, and avoidance of contact sports for 6–8 weeks.
- For severe pharyngitis, consider gonorrhea and treat per STD/STI protocol.

BPPV   10 mg twice a day for 5 days

32

BLEPHARITIS

Common organisms: S. aureus, coagulase-negative staphylococci

Note: Antibiotics are usually not necessary unless local care is unsuccessful. There are various antibiotic ointment options. Apply to lid margin, up to four times a day for up to one month.

- Bacitracin ophthalmic ointment
- Erythromycin ophthalmic ointment
- Sulfacetamide ophthalmic ointment

PEARLS

- Lid hygiene: apply warm compresses to closed lid for 5–10 min two to four times a day to loosen crusts, and then wash/massage lids with a cotton swab soaked in a mixture of baby shampoo and water (1:1 mix).

CONJUNCTIVITIS

Common organisms: Viral, S. aureus, S. pneumoniae, H. influenzae, Pseudomonas spp., N. gonorrhea, C. trachomatis

- Bacterial conjunctivitis (non-gonococcal, non-chlamydial)
- Polymyxin B/trimethoprim sol. 1–2 drops every 3–6 hours for 7–10 days
- Erythromycin 0.5% ophthalmic ointment ½ inch to conjunctival sac four times daily for 5–7 days
- Sulfacetamide 10% sol. ophthalmic drops 1–2 drops every 6 hours for 5–7 days
- Levofloxacin 0.5% sol. 1–2 drops every 2 hours while awake for 2 days, **THEN** every 4–8 hours for 5 days
- Moxifloxacin 0.5% sol. 1–2 drops every 2 hours while awake for 2 days, **THEN** every 4–8 hours for 5 days
- Gatifloxacin 0.5% sol. 1–2 drops every 2 hours while awake for 2 days, **THEN** every 4–8 hours for 5 days

Gonococcal Conjunctivitis

- Ceftriaxone 1 g IM/IV (50 mg/kg IM/IV – max dose 125 mg IM) for 1 dose **PLUS**
  - Azithromycin 1g (20 mg/kg) PO once **OR**
  - Doxycycline 100 mg two times daily PO for 7 days

EYE

33

Chlamydial Conjunctivitis
- Azithromycin 1 g (20 mg/kg) PO once
- Doxycycline 100 mg two times daily PO for 7 days

Newborn
- Ceftriaxone 50 mg/kg IM/IV (max dose 125 mg) once *AND* erythromycin 12.5 mg/kg PO four times daily for 14 days

PEARLS
- The majority of conjunctivitis is viral and does not require treatment.
- Eye drops preferred for adults, and ointments for children.
- Fluoroquinolones are first-line treatment for contact lens wearers, but are the most expensive option.
- Discontinue contact lens use for at least 2 weeks, and do not resume until infection has cleared. Discard lens case, eye drops, and disposable lenses. If lenses are not disposable, reuse only after overnight disinfection.

CORNEAL ABRASION

Non-Contact Lens User (treatment duration: 3–5 days)
Common organisms: *Staphylococcus spp., Streptococcus spp.*
- Erythromycin ophthalmic ointment: apply four times daily
- Sulfacetamide 10% ophthalmic ointment: apply four times daily
- Sulfacetamide 10% sol. instill 1–2 drops four times daily
- Ciprofloxacin 0.3% sol. instill 1–2 drops four times daily
- Ofloxacin 0.3% sol. instill 1–2 drops four times daily

Contact Lens User
Common organisms: *Pseudomonas spp.*
- Levofloxacin 0.5% sol. instill 1–2 drops every 2 hours while awake for 2 days, *THEN* every 4–8 hours for 5 days
- Moxifloxacin 0.5% sol. instill 1–2 drops every 2 hours while awake for 2 days, *THEN* every 4–8 hours for 5 days
- Gatifloxacin 0.5% sol. instill 1–2 drops every 2 hours while awake for 2 days, *THEN* every 4–8 hours for 5 days
- Gentamicin 0.3% sol instill 1–2 drops six times daily for 5 days
- Tobramycin 0.3% sol instill 1–2 drops four times daily for 5 days

PEARLS

- Antibiotic treatment is recommended for contact lens users.
- In recurrent abrasion, ointment is the preferred method of treatment.
- The use of ointment is favored in children.
- Untreated corneal abrasions can progress to corneal ulcers.
- Contact lens users need to discontinue use of lenses and have 24-hour follow up with ophthalmology.
- Due to increasing first- and second-generation fluoroquinolone resistance, use of third- and fourth-generation fluoroquinolones is recommended for contact lens users.
- Avoid the use of topical corticosteroids and eye patches in patients with corneal abrasions.
- Address tetanus status.

ORBITAL CELLULITIS

Common organisms: *Streptococcus spp., Staphylococcus spp., H. influenzae,* anaerobes

- Vancomycin 15–20 mg/kg IV two times daily (15 mg/kg IV four times daily) **PLUS**
  - Ampicillin/sulbactam 3 g (50 mg/kg) IV four times daily **OR**
  - Ceftriaxone 2 g (100 mg/kg) IV once daily **OR**
  - Levofloxacin 750 mg IV once daily **AND** metronidazole 500 mg IV three times daily **OR**
  - Clindamycin 600 mg IV three times daily (10 mg/kg IV four times daily)

PEARLS

- Orbital cellulitis is associated with limited or painful extra-ocular motion.
- Proptosis, visual changes, or vision loss can occur.
- Headache, fever, globe displacement, meningeal signs or cranial nerve deficits may also exist.
- CT scan of orbits/sinuses may help differentiate from periorbital cellulitis.
- Consider MRI/MRV or CT venography for detection of cavernous sinus thrombosis.
- Consider fungal etiologies (mucormycoses and aspergillus) in refractory cases or patients with immunodeficiency.

PERIORBITAL CELLULITIS

Common organisms: *Staphylococcus spp., Streptococcus spp., anaerobes,* historically *H. influenzae*

Outpatient

- Clindamycin 450 mg PO three times daily (10 mg/kg PO four times daily) for 7–10 days
- Cephalexin 500 mg (25 mg/kg) PO four times daily for 5 days *AND* TMP/SMX (DS) 2 tablets (5 mg/kg) PO two times daily

Inpatient

- Follow guidelines for orbital cellulitis (page 35).

PEARLS

- CT scan of orbits/sinuses helps to differentiate from orbital cellulitis.
- Indications for CT scan of orbits/sinuses include inability to assess vision secondary to edema, proptosis, ophthalmoplegia, change in visual acuity, bilateral periorbital edema, CNS symptoms, and no improvement after 24 hrs of outpatient therapy.
- Pediatric patients (<1 yr) or severe cases of periorbital cellulitis should be admitted for IV antibiotics and treated with guidelines for orbital cellulitis.

APPENDICITIS

Common organisms: *Enterobacteriaceae (E. coli, Klebsiella spp., Proteus spp.), Bacteroides spp.*

Simple Appendicitis, Pediatric
- Ertapenem 7.5 mg/kg IV two times daily (max dose 1 g/day)
- Piperacillin-tazobactam 100 mg/kg IV three times daily
- Gentamicin 2.5 mg/kg IV three times daily **PLUS**
  - Metronidazole 7.5 mg/kg IV four times daily **OR**
  - Clindamycin 10 mg/kg IV three times daily
- Metronidazole 7.5 mg/kg IV four times daily **PLUS**
  - Ceftriaxone 50 mg/kg IV once daily **OR**
  - Cefotaxime 50 mg/kg IV four times daily

Simple Appendicitis, Adult
- Cefoxitin 2 g IV four times daily
- Ertapenem 1 g IV once daily
- Moxifloxacin 400 mg IV once daily
- Ticarcillin/clavulanate 3.1 g IV four times daily
- Metronidazole 500 mg IV three times daily **PLUS**
  - Ceftriaxone 1 g IV once daily **OR**
  - Cefotaxime 1 g IV three times daily

Complicated Appendicitis (gangrenous, perforated, abscess or phlegmon)

Adults and Pediatrics
- Imipenem/cilastatin 500 mg (25 mg/kg) IV four times daily
- Piperacillin/tazobactam 4.5 g (100 mg/kg) IV three times daily
- Metronidazole 500 mg IV three times daily (7.5 mg/kg IV four times daily) **PLUS**
  - Cefepime 2g (50 mg/kg) IV two times daily **OR**
  - Ceftazidime 2g (50 mg/kg) IV three times daily **OR**
  - Ciprofloxacin 400 mg IV two times daily **OR**
  - Levofloxacin 750 mg IV once daily

[handwritten notes:]
lansoprazole
H pylori 10-14 days 30
PPI : omeprazole 30 mg twice daily
amoxicillin 1g twice daily ↑ or metronidazole 500 mg twice daily
clarithromycin 500mg twice daily ↑

PEARLS

- The antibiotic regimen listed for complicated appendicitis is also recommended in the following situations:
  - Delay in initial intervention (>24 hrs)
  - Immunocompromised/suppressed state
  - Poor nutritional status/low albumin level
  - Significant cardiovascular disease/multiple comorbidities
  - Healthcare-associated infections (e.g., recent hospitalization, antibiotics, extended care facility residents, etc.)
  - High Apache II scores

CHOLANGITIS

Common organisms: *E. Coli, Klebsiella spp., Pseudomonas spp., Enterobacter spp., Enterococcus spp., Bacteroides spp., Clostridium spp., Streptococcus spp.*

Mild to Moderate Disease

- Cefazolin 1 g IV three times daily
- Ceftriaxone 1 g IV once daily
- Cefuroxime 1.5 g IV three times daily
- Ciprofloxacin 400 mg IV two times daily
- Levofloxacin 750 mg IV once daily
- Moxifloxacin 400 mg IV once daily

Severe/Life-Threatening Disease

- Metronidazole 500 mg IV three times daily *PLUS*
  - Ceftazidime 2 g IV three times daily *OR*
  - Cefepime 2 g IV three times daily *OR*
  - Aztreonam 2 g IV three times daily
- Piperacillin/tazobactam 4.5 g IV three times daily
- Imipenem/cilastatin 500 mg IV four times daily

PEARLS

- For severe/life-threatening infection must cover empirically for *Pseudomonas spp.* and *Enterococcus spp.*
- Consider *Enterococcus spp.* coverage for those with healthcare-associated infections, post-operative, recent cephalosporin exposure, and immunocompromised patients.
- Consider adding vancomycin for severe/life threatening infection or when aztreonam is utilized.

38

DIVERTICULITIS

Common organisms: *Enterobacteriaceae, Bacteroides spp., Enterococcus spp.*

Outpatient Therapy (treatment duration: 7–10 days)
- Metronidazole 500 mg PO three times daily *PLUS*
  - Ciprofloxacin 500 mg PO two times daily *OR*
  - Levofloxacin 750 mg PO once daily
- Moxifloxacin 400 mg PO once daily

Inpatient Therapy, Mild to Moderate Disease
- Metronidazole 500 mg IV three times daily *PLUS*
  - Ciprofloxacin 400 mg IV two times daily *OR*
  - Levofloxacin 750 mg IV once daily *OR*
  - Aztreonam 2 g IV three times daily *OR*
  - Ceftriaxone 1 g IV once daily
- Ertapenem 1 g IV once daily
- Moxifloxacin 400 mg IV once daily

Inpatient Therapy, Severe Disease
- Imipenem/cilastatin 500 mg IV four times daily
- Piperacillin/tazobactam 4.5 g IV three times daily
- Vancomycin 15–20 mg/kg IV two times daily *AND* metronidazole 500 mg IV three times daily *PLUS*
  - Ciprofloxacin 400 mg IV two times daily *OR*
  - Levofloxacin 750 mg IV once daily *OR*
  - Aztreonam 2 g IV three times daily

PEARLS
- Consider enterococcal coverage: healthcare-associated infections, post-operative, recent cephalosporin exposure, immunocompromised patients (e.g., piperacillin/tazobactam).
- Consider adding vancomycin for severe/life-threatening infection.

INFECTIOUS DIARRHEA

Bacteria: *Campylobacter jejuni, C. difficile, E. coli, L. monocytogenes, Salmonella spp., Shigella, Vibrio cholerae, Yersinia enterocolitica*

Viruses: *Adenovirus, Astrovirus, Rotavirus, Norovirus (Norwalk)*

Protozoa: *Cryptosporidium, Cyclospora, Entamoeba histolytica, Giardia*

PEARLS

- Antibiotic therapy is **not** required in most cases since the illness is usually self-limited. Consider empiric therapy for traveler's diarrhea, diarrhea that lasts longer than 10–14 days, or for febrile diarrhea.

Empiric Therapy (treatment duration: 3–5 days)

- Ciprofloxacin 500 mg PO two times daily
- Levofloxacin 500 mg PO once daily
- TMP/SMX (DS) 1 tablet (5 mg/kg) PO two times daily

Campylobacter Jejuni (treatment duration: 3–5 days)

- Ciprofloxacin 500 mg PO two times daily
- Azithromycin 500 mg (10 mg/kg) PO once daily for 3 days

Clostridium Difficile

- See Pseudomembranous Colitis section (page 41).

E. Coli 0157:H7

- Antibiotic treatment is not generally recommended as it may increase the risk of hemolytic uremic syndrome.

Salmonella (Non-Typhoid) (treatment duration: 5–7 days, 14 days for immunocompromised patients)

- Routine treatment is not recommended.
- May consider treatment for age <6 months >50 years, or has prostheses, valvular heart disease, severe atherosclerosis, malignancy, sickle cell, AAA, or uremia.
  - Ciprofloxacin 500 mg PO two times daily
  - Levofloxacin 500 mg PO once daily
  - Ceftriaxone 2 g (100 mg/kg) IV once daily
  - TMP/SMX (DS) 1 tablet (5 mg/kg) PO two times daily

Shigella (treatment duration: 3–5 days unless otherwise noted; 7–10 days for immunocompromised patients)

- Ciprofloxacin 500 mg PO two times daily
- Levofloxacin 500 mg PO once daily
- TMP/SMX (DS) 1 tablet (5 mg/kg) PO two times daily for 5 days
- Azithromycin 500 mg (10 mg/kg) PO daily for 5 days

Vibrio Cholerae

- Doxycycline 300 mg PO once
- TMP/SMX (DS) 1 tablet (5 mg/kg) PO two times daily for 3 days
- Ciprofloxacin 1 g PO once

Yersinia Enterocolitica (treatment duration: 3 days)

- Antibiotics are not usually required unless bacteremia is present.
  - Ciprofloxacin 500 mg PO two times daily
  - Levofloxacin 500 mg PO once daily
  - TMP/SMX (DS) 1 tablet (5 mg/kg) PO two times daily

Entamoeba Histolytica

- Metronidazole 750 mg PO three times daily for 5–10 days *PLUS*
  - Paromomycin 500 mg three times daily for 7 days *OR*
  - Iodoquinol 650 mg three times daily for 20 days

Giardia Lambia

- Metronidazole 250 mg PO three times daily for 7–10 days
- Tinidazole 2 g PO once

PSEUDOMEMBRANOUS COLITIS (HEALTHCARE-ASSOCIATED DIARRHEAL ILLNESS)

Common organism: *C. difficile* (treatment duration: 10–14 days)

Initial Episode, Mild-Moderate Disease — WBC < 15,000 cells/mL *AND* serum creatinine level <1.5 times the premorbid level

- Metronidazole 500 mg PO three times daily

Initial Episode, Severe Disease — WBC >15,000 cells/mL *OR* serum creatinine level >1.5 times the premorbid level, albumin <2.5 g/dl

- Vancomycin 125 mg PO four times daily

41

Initial Episode, Severe, Complicated Disease (hypotension, shock, ileus or megacolon)
- Metronidazole 500 mg IV three times daily *AND* vancomycin 500 mg PO four times daily
- For ileus, consider adding vancomycin 500 mg in 100 ml saline four times daily as retention enema

First Recurrence
- Same treatment as initial episode

Second Recurrence
- Vancomycin in pulse or tapered dosing

PEARLS
- Avoid medications that decrease intestinal motility.
- Oral medications are preferred over IV.
- Consult infectious disease for post-treatment relapse.
- Consider surgical consult for colectomy in severe complicated disease.

PERITONITIS/PERFORATED VISCOUS/ INTRA-ABDOMINAL ABSCESS

Common organisms: Typically *polymicrobial* involving *enteric gram-negative aerobic, facultative bacilli, and enteric gram-positive streptococci*

Mild to Moderate Disease
- Metronidazole 500 mg IV three times daily (7.5 mg/kg IV four times daily) *PLUS*
  - Ciprofloxacin 400 mg IV two times daily *OR*
  - Levofloxacin 750 mg IV once daily *OR*
  - Cefazolin 1 g (30 mg/kg) IV three times daily *OR*
  - Ceftriaxone 1g (50 mg/kg) IV once daily *OR*
  - Cefuroxime 1g (50 mg/kg) IV/IM three times daily
- Moxifloxacin 400 mg IV once daily
- Cefoxitin 2 g (25 mg/kg) IV four times daily

Severe, Life-Threatening Disease
- Piperacillin/tazobactam 4.5 g (80 mg/kg) IV three times daily
- Metronidazole 500 mg IV three times daily (7.5 mg/kg IV four times daily) **AND** cefepime 2 g (50 mg/kg) IV two times daily
- Imipenem/cilastatin 500 mg IV four times daily (25 mg/kg IV four times daily)
- Vancomycin 15–20 mg/kg IV two times daily (10 mg/kg IV four times daily) **AND** aztreonam 2 g (30 mg/kg) IV three times daily **AND** metronidazole 500 mg IV three times daily (7.5 mg/kg IV four times daily)

PERITONEAL DIALYSIS-RELATED PERITONITIS

Common organisms: *Staphylococcus spp. (including MRSA), Streptococcus spp., Pseudomonas spp., Klebsiella spp., Enterobacter spp., polymicrobial, anaerobes, Candida spp., Mycobacterium spp.*

PEARLS
- Empirically cover for both gram-positive and gram-negative organisms.
- Consider early nephrology and/or ID consult, as intraperitoneal administration of antibiotics may be needed.
- CAPD: Greater than 100 WBC/mm^3 in the peritoneal fluid, with neutrophilic predominance.

INTRAPERITONEAL ROUTE
Gram-Positive Coverage
- Cefazolin 15 mg/kg per exchange once daily
- If MRSA suspected: vancomycin 15–30 mg/kg every 5–7 days

AND

Gram-Negative Coverage
- Ceftazidime 1000–1500 mg per exchange once daily
- Cefepime 1000 mg per exchange once daily
- Gentamicin 0.6 mg/kg per exchange once daily

IV ROUTE
Gram-Positive Coverage (MRSA coverage)
- Vancomycin 15–20 mg/kg IV
- Linezolid 600 mg IV
- Daptomycin 4–6 mg/kg IV

AND

Gram-Negative Coverage
- Ceftazidime 2 g IV
- Imipenem/cilastatin 125–250 mg IV
- Aztreonam 500 mg IV
- Levofloxacin 750 mg IV
- Ciprofloxacin 400 mg IV

PEARLS
- Consider treatment for fungal peritonitis if patient has received recent antibiotic treatment for bacterial peritonitis.
- Intraperitoneal administration is preferred treatment.

SPONTANEOUS BACTERIAL PERITONITIS

Common organisms: *E. coli, Klebsiella spp., Streptococcus spp., Enterobacter spp., Staphylococcus spp., polymicrobial (secondary peritonitis), anaerobes (secondary peritonitis)*
- Ceftriaxone 1 g IV once daily
- Ciprofloxacin 400 mg IV two times daily
- Levofloxacin 750 mg IV once daily
- Moxifloxacin 400 mg IV once daily
- Pipercillin/tazobactam 4.5 g IV three times daily

Prior Quinolone Prophylaxis
- *ADD* Vancomycin 15–20 mg/kg IV two times daily to above

PEARLS
- SBP: Greater than 250 PMN/mm^3 in the peritoneal fluid.
- Consider addition of 1.5 g albumin/kg body weight in setting of suspected SBP *AND* serum creatinine >1 mg/dL, blood urea nitrogen >30 mg/dL, or total bilirubin >4 mg/dL.

44

BALANITIS

Common organisms: *Candida spp.,* occasionally *Group B Streptococcus,*
anaerobes

- Clotrimazole 1% applied two times daily until symptoms resolve
- Miconazole 2% applied two times daily until symptoms resolve
- Severe symptoms: fluconazole 150 mg PO once
- Suspected *anaerobes*: metronidazole 500 mg two times daily for 7 days
- Suspected *Staph* or *Strep*: cephalexin 500 mg PO two times daily for
  7 days **OR** clindamycin 450 mg PO three times daily for 7 days

PEARLS

- Balanitis that persists despite treatment mandates urologic follow up
  and possible biopsy.
- Consider new diagnosis of diabetes.
- Consider reactive arthritis, herpes virus, trichomonas, and syphilis.
- Sitz baths with daily gentle retraction of the foreskin are recommended.
- Screen for STD/STI and treat partners.

ENDOMETRITIS

Moderate to Severe Disease

Common organisms: Often polymicrobial (including *anaerobes*), including
C. trachomatis and *M. hominis*

- Clindamycin 900 mg IV three times daily **AND** gentamicin 5–7 mg/kg IV
  once daily
- Doxycycline 100 mg IV/PO two times daily **PLUS**
  - Cefoxitin 2 g IV four times daily **OR**
  - Ampicillin/sulbactam 3 g IV four times daily

Mild Disease: Limited to Decidua and Myometrium

- Ceftriaxone 250 mg IM **PLUS**
  - Doxycycline 100 mg PO two times daily for 14 days **WITH OR
    WITHOUT**
    - Metronidazole 500 mg PO two times daily for 14 days

GU

45

PEARLS

- Early postpartum (from 24 hrs to 1 week) infection usually occurs after C-section.
- Cesarean delivery more likely to have anaerobic infection.
- Late postpartum (1 to 6 weeks) infection usually occurs after vaginal delivery; can present as postpartum hemorrhage.
- Intrapartum treatment should be initiated for infection during delivery.
- Tetracyclines are not recommended in nursing mothers.
- Consider removal of intrauterine devices.

EPIDIDYMITIS/ORCHITIS

Common organisms: Age <35: *N. gonorrhea, C. trachomatis.*
Age >35: *Pseudomonas spp., E. coli*

STD Suspected

- Doxycycline 100 mg PO two times daily for 10 days *AND* ceftriaxone 250 mg IM once
- If PCN allergic: azithromycin 2 g PO once

STD Not Suspected (treatment duration: 10 days)

- Levofloxacin 500 mg PO once daily
- If associated with prostatitis, continue treatment for 21 days.

PEARLS

- Rest, ice, NSAIDs, and scrotal support are important adjuncts.
- The sexual partner should also be treated.
- CDC recommends test of cure 7 days after treatment in instances where ceftriaxone was not utilized.
- Consider testicular torsion; Doppler ultrasound is helpful in differentiating epididymitis from torsion.
- Prehn's sign (decreased pain with scrotal elevation) is not reliable in distinguishing epididymitis from torsion.
- Consider mumps for isolated orchitis.

PROSTATITIS

Common organisms: *E. coli.* Consider *N. gonorrhea* and *C. trachomatis* coverage if STD/STI suspected

STD/STI Not Suspected (treatment duration: 14–28)
- Ciprofloxacin 500 mg PO two times daily
- Levofloxacin 500 mg PO once daily
- TMP/SMX (DS) 1 tablet PO two times daily

STD/STI Suspected (treatment duration: 14 days)
- Doxycycline 100 mg PO two times daily *AND* ceftriaxone 250 mg IM once
- Ciprofloxacin 500 mg PO two times daily (avoid where quinolone-resistent gonorrhea is prevalent)

For Severe Infection (bacteremia, sepsis, or suspected prostatic abscess)
- Ciprofloxacin 400 mg IV two times daily
- Levofloxacin 500 mg IV once daily
- Ceftriaxone 2 g IV once daily

PEARLS
- Total length of therapy should be at least 28 days if there is concern for chronic prostatitis.
- *E. coli* causes 75–80% of infections.
- Chronic bacterial prostatitis is associated with urethral catheters or instrumentation.
- Urine gram-stain and culture recommended in all men suspected of acute prostatitis.

SEXUAL ASSAULT STD PROPHYLAXIS

Common organisms: *C. trachomatis, N. gonorrhea, Trichomonas spp., Hepatitis B, HIV, Tetanus*
- Ceftriaxone 250 mg IM once *AND* metronidazole 2 g PO once *PLUS*
  — Azithromycin 1 g PO once *OR*
  — Doxycycline 100 mg PO two times daily for 7 days
- HBV/HIV exposure: See *Occupational Post-Exposure Prophylaxis (PEP)* chapter.

47

PEARLS

- Azithromycin 2 g PO once may be substituted for ceftriaxone in penicillin-allergic patients; test of cure one week after treatment is recommended.
- Serologic testing for syphilis, HBV, HCV, and HIV also recommended by the CDC.
- Consider pregnancy prophylaxis up to 5 days post exposure.
- Consider tetanus booster if indicated.

BACTERIAL VAGINOSIS

Common organisms: *Gardnerella spp., polymicrobial* (treatment duration: 7 days unless otherwise noted)

- Metronidazole 500 mg PO two times daily
- Clindamycin 300 mg PO two times daily
- Metronidazole vaginal gel 0.75% one applicator vaginally daily or nightly for 5 days
- Clindamycin vaginal cream 2% one applicator vaginally daily or nightly for 7 days

PEARLS

- No need to treat partner.
- May substitute tinidazole 2 g PO once daily for 2 days.
- Pregnancy
  - Oral regimens generally preferred in pregnancy.

VULVOVAGINAL CANDIDIASIS

Intravaginal Therapy for Uncomplicated Candidal Vaginitis (preparations available OTC)

- Clotrimazole 1% cream one applicator vaginally for 7–14 nights **OR** 2% cream one applicator vaginally for 3 nights
- Miconazole 2% cream one applicator vaginally for 7 nights **OR** 4% cream one applicator vaginally for 3 nights
- Miconazole 100 mg one suppository vaginally for 7 nights **OR** one 200 mg suppository vaginally for 3 nights
- Tioconazole 6.5% ointment one applicator vaginally once
- Butoconazole 2% cream one applicator vaginally for 3 nights (do not use during first trimester of pregnancy)

Intravaginal Therapy for Uncomplicated Candidal Vaginitis (prescription)

- Nystatin 100,000–unit vaginal tablet, one tablet vaginally for 14 nights
- Terconazole 80 mg one suppository vaginally for 3 nights *OR* 0.8% cream vaginally for 3 nights

Oral Therapy for Vulvovaginal Candidiasis

- Fluconazole 150 mg PO once (may repeat in 72 hours if symptoms persist)

PEARLS

- Only topical imidazole (clotrimazole, miconazole) therapy, applied for 7 days, is recommended in pregnancy.
- If symptoms persist or recur within 2 months, patients should seek medical follow up.
- Topically applied azole drugs are more effective than nystatin.

TRICHOMONIASIS

- Metronidazole 2 g PO once *OR* 500 mg PO two times daily for 7 days
- Tinidazole 2 g PO once

PEARLS

- The treatment of asymptomatic pregnant women is controversial, risks/benefits should be discussed with the patient; metronidazole is the preferred treatment for symptomatic patients.
- Sexual partners should be treated with metronidazole 500 mg PO two times daily for 7 days *OR* tinidazole 2 g PO once.
- Avoid breastfeeding and alcohol use until 24 hours after the last dose of metronidazole, or 72 hours after the last dose of tinidazole.

URETHRITIS/CERVICITIS

Co-infection is common with gonorrhea and chlamydia; treat for both.

Common organisms: *C. trachomatis, U. urealyticum, M. genitalium, Trichomonas spp., HSV*

- Ceftriaxone 250 mg IM once *PLUS*
  - Azithromycin 1 g PO once *OR*
  - Doxycycline 100 mg PO two times daily for 7 days

If severe penicillin or cephalosporin allergy:

- Azithromycin 2 g PO once
- Test of cure recommended 7 days after treatment

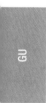

PEARLS

- Treat partners or known contacts within past 60 days (or the most recent partner if contact was >60 days prior). Patients should abstain from intercourse until 7 days after therapy is initiated *AND* symptom resolution *AND* partners have been treated.
- Fluoroquinolones are no longer recommended for treatment of gonococcal urethritis/cervicitis due to rising levels of resistance among *N. gonorrhea* isolates. Similar resistance is emerging for azithromycin and cefixime.
- Consider testing patient for other STDs such as HIV and syphilis.
- Consider treatment with metronidazole for *Trichomonas spp.* and/or bacterial vaginosis infection, especially in resistant cases.
- In pregnancy, repeat testing 3 weeks after completion of therapy is indicated.

PELVIC INFLAMMATORY DISEASE

Common organisms: *N. gonorrhea, C. trachomatis, S. agalactiae, G. vaginalis,* enteric gram-negative rods, *anaerobes*

Outpatient

- Doxycycline 100 mg PO two times daily for 14 days *AND* ceftriaxone 250 mg IM once
- **CONSIDER ADDING:** Metronidazole 500 mg PO two times daily for 14 days

Inpatient

- Doxycycline 100 mg IV/PO two times daily **PLUS**
  — Cefoxitin 2 g IV four times daily **OR**
  — Cefotetan 2 g IV two times daily **OR**
- Clindamycin 900 mg IV three times daily **AND** gentamicin 5 mg/kg IV daily

PEARLS

- Fluoroquinolones are no longer recommended, due to rising levels of resistance among *N. gonorrhea* isolates (may be considered for outpatient regimen if true cephalosporin allergy).
- Consider admission for
  — Suspected TOA or pelvic abscess
  — Pregnancy
  — Nausea, vomiting, high fever, or failure of outpatient therapy
  — Any patient if compliance or follow up is questionable
- Consider testing the patient for syphilis, HIV.
- Treat partners or known contacts within past 60 days (or the most recent partner if contact was >60 days prior). Patients should abstain from intercourse until therapy is completed **AND** symptom resolution **AND** partners have been treated.

HERPES SIMPLEX VIRUS

First Episode (treatment duration: 7–10 days)

- Acyclovir 400 mg PO three times daily
- Valacyclovir 1 g PO two times daily
- Famciclovir 250 mg PO three times daily

Recurrent Episode

- Acyclovir 800 mg PO two times daily for 5 days
- Acyclovir 800 mg PO three times daily for 2 days
- Valacyclovir 500 mg PO two times daily for 3 days
- Valacyclovir 1 g PO once daily for 5 days
- Famciclovir 1 g PO two times daily for 1 day

Suppressive Therapy

- Acyclovir 400 mg PO two times daily
- Famciclovir 250 mg PO two times daily
- Valacyclovir 1 g PO once daily

GU

Episodic (First or Recurrent) Therapy for HIV-Positive (treatment duration: 5–10 days)

- Acyclovir 400 mg PO three times daily
- Famciclovir 500 mg PO two times daily
- Valacyclovir 1 g PO two times daily

Suppressive Therapy for HIV-Positive

- Acyclovir 400 mg PO three times daily
- Acyclovir 800 mg PO two times daily
- Famciclovir 500 mg PO two times daily
- Valacyclovir 500 mg PO two times daily

Severe Disease or Complicated Course (disseminated infection, pneumonitis, hepatitis, meningitis, or encephalitis)

- Acyclovir 10 mg/kg IV three times daily (acyclovir dosing is based on *ideal* body weight, not *actual* body weight)

SYPHILIS

Common organism: *T. pallidum*

Primary/Secondary/Early Latent Syphilis

- Benzathine penicillin G 2.4 million units IM once
- Doxycycline 100 mg PO two times daily for 14 days

Tertiary Syphilis/Late Latent Syphilis/Syphilis of Unknown Duration

- Benzathine penicillin G 2.4 million units IM once a week for 3 weeks
- Doxycycline 100 mg PO two times daily for 28 days

Neurosyphilis (including ocular syphilis)

- Penicillin G 3–4 million units IV six times daily for 10–14 days

PEARLS

- Counsel patients on the potential Jarisch-Herxheimer reaction (rigors, fever, hypotension).
- Very limited data on efficacy of regimens other than penicillin.
- Treatment during pregnancy should be the penicillin regimen appropriate for the stage of syphilis.
- **Early latent** = latent disease, acquired in the past year. **Late latent** = latent disease, possibly or probably acquired more than one year ago.

- Pregnant and neurosyphilis patients allergic to penicillin should be desensitized and treated with penicillin.
- Recommend LP for all HIV-positive patients with syphilis.

URINARY TRACT INFECTION (UTI)/CYSTITIS

Uncomplicated UTI, Adult

Common organisms: *E. coli, S. saprophyticus, Enterococcus spp., Klebsiella spp.*

Empiric Agents
- Nitrofurantoin 100 mg PO two times daily for 5 days (avoid if early pyelonephritis suspected)
- TMP/SMX (DS) 1 tablet PO two times daily for 3 days (avoid if used for UTI in previous 6 months)
  - If local *E. coli* resistance >20% to TMP/SMX, use alternative agent
- β-lactam (treatment duration: 3–7 days)
  - Cephalexin 500 mg PO two times daily
  - Cefpodoxime proxetil 100 mg PO two times daily
- Fosfomycin 3 g once
- Fluoroquinolone (treatment duration: 3 days)
  - Ciprofloxacin 250 mg PO two times daily for 3 days
  - Levofloxacin 250 mg PO once daily for 3 days

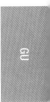

If Pregnant (treatment duration: 7 days)
- Nitrofurantoin 100 mg PO two times daily
- Cephalexin 500 mg PO two times daily

Complicated UTI (nosocomial, obstruction, catheters, reflux), Adult

Common organisms: *E. coli, Pseudomonas spp., Enterococcus spp., Klebsiella spp., Serratia spp., Citrobacter spp.*
- Ciprofloxacin 500 mg PO two times daily for 7 days **OR** 400 mg IV two times daily
- Levofloxacin 750 mg IV/PO once daily for 5 days
- Ampicillin 1 g IV four times daily **AND** gentamicin 5 mg/kg IV daily
- Cefepime 2 g IV two times daily
- Imipenem/cilastatin 500 mg IV four times daily (reserve carbapenems for suspected ESBLs)

2015 EMRA Antibiotic Guide

Uncomplicated UTI, Pediatric (treatment duration: 5 days if >2 years and first UTI; 7–14 days if has a history of UTI's, or age <2 yrs)

- Cefixime 8 mg/kg PO once daily
- Amoxicillin/clavulanic acid 10 mg/kg PO three times daily
- TMP/SMX 5 mg/kg (TMP-based) PO two times daily

Complicated UTI (nosocomial, obstruction, catheters, reflux), Pediatric

Note: Begin with IV therapy and switch to PO once afebrile for 48–72 hours

- Ceftriaxone 100 mg/kg IV once daily
- Cefotaxime 50 mg/kg IV three times daily
- Gentamicin 2.5 mg/kg IV three times daily

PEARLS

- Local resistance patterns vary widely; recommend against agents that have a <20% resistance to *E.coli*.
- Treat women with asymptomatic bacteriuria only if they are pregnant.
- Rule out vaginitis, chlamydia, gonorrhea, and HSV in sexually active patients.
- Gram stain and culture for pediatric or complicated infections.
- For analgesia, may use phenazopyridine 200 mg PO three times daily for 2 days (adults); 4 mg/kg three times daily for 2 days (children 6–12 years old).

PYELONEPHRITIS

Common organisms: *E. coli, Enterococcus spp., Klebsiella spp., Proteus spp., S. saprophyticus*

Outpatient, Adults

Note: If local fluroquinolone resistance >10%, consider one-time dosing of ceftriaxone 1 g IV **OR** an aminoglycoside 5–7 mg/kg pending susceptibility; follow with oral regimen below.

- TMP/SMX (DS) 1 tablet PO two times daily for 14 days (if known susceptibility)
- Ciprofloxacin 500 mg PO two times daily for 7 days
- Levofloxacin 750 mg PO once daily for 5 days
- Cefpodoxime 200 mg PO two times daily for 10–14 days
- Cephalexin 500 mg PO three times daily for 10–14 days

Inpatient, Adult

Note: Begin with IV therapy and switch to PO once afebrile for 24–48 hours.

If Not Suspecting Enterococcal Infection

- Ciprofloxacin 400 mg IV two times daily
- Levofloxacin 750 mg IV once daily
- Ceftriaxone 1 g IV once daily
- Cefepime 2 g IV two times daily
- Imipenem 500 mg four times daily
- Aztreonam 2 g IV three times daily (if beta-lactam allergic)

If Suspected or Known Enterococcal Infection

- Ampicillin 2 g IV four times daily *AND* gentamicin 1 mg/kg IV three times daily
- Piperacillin-tazobactam 4.5 g IV three times daily
- Ampicillin-sulbactam 3 g IV four times daily

Inpatient, Pediatric

Note: Begin with IV therapy, and switch to PO once afebrile for 48–72 hours.

- Ceftriaxone 100 mg/kg IV once daily
- Cefotaxime 50 mg/kg IV three times daily
- Ampicillin 25 mg/kg IV four times daily *AND* gentamicin 2.5 mg/kg IV three times daily

PEARLS

- In general, admit all pregnant patients with pyelonephritis.
- Patients with hypotension/shock, recurrent pyelonephritis, or persistent symptoms after 3 days of treatment should be imaged to rule out stone or perinephric abscess.
- Pediatric patients should have urologic follow up to rule out urinary tract malformations.

GU

BRONCHITIS

PEARLS

- The vast majority of cases are caused by viruses.
- Antibiotics are not considered the mainstay of treatment, and may increase adverse events and antimicrobial-resistance.
- Antitussives and bronchodilators may be helpful in adults.
- For prolonged cough (>10 days), antibiotic treatment may be occasionally warranted.
- Consider pertussis in patients with prolonged cough, and inquire about close contacts with viral symptoms.
- Mycoplasma pneumonia may cause prolonged cough in children >5 years of age.
- Treat those at high risk of serious complications due to pre-existing comorbidity (heart, lung, renal, liver, neuromuscular disease, or immunosuppression).
  - See AECB for antimicrobial options (below).

ACUTE EXACERBATION OF CHRONIC BRONCHITIS (AECB)

Common organisms: *Viral, C. pneumoniae, M. pneumoniae, H. influenzae, M. catarrhalis, S. pneumoniae, Pseudomonas spp.*

Outpatient (treatment duration: 5–10 days unless otherwise noted)

- Azithromycin 500 mg PO once daily for day 1, **THEN** 250 mg PO once daily for days 2 through 5
- Doxycycline 100 mg PO two times daily
- Cefuroxime 500 mg PO two times daily
- TMP/SMX (DS) 1 tablet PO two times daily
- Amoxicillin/clavulanate 875 mg PO two times daily
- Levofloxacin 750 mg PO once daily for 5 days
- Moxifloxacin 400 mg PO once daily for 5 days

Inpatient

- Azithromycin 500 mg IV once daily
- Ceftriaxone 1 g IV once daily
- Levofloxacin 750 mg PO/IV once daily
- Moxifloxacin 400 mg PO/IV once daily

PEARLS

- Cardinal symptoms of AECB = increased dyspnea, increased sputum volume, increased sputum purulence.
- 50–70% of AECB are bacterial; however, it may not be necessary to treat mild exacerbations (with only 1 cardinal symptom) with antibiotics.
- Adjuncts for COPD exacerbations and AECB include inhaled anticholinergic bronchodilators, oral corticosteroids.
- Consider combination therapy in suspected *Pseudomonas* spp infection.

INFLUENZA

PEARLS

- Amantadine or rimantadine should not be used for the treatment or prevention of influenza.
- Treatment may decrease duration of illness by 1–3 days if started within 48 hours of symptom onset.
- Little to no benefit in treatment after 48 hours of illness in uncomplicated cases.
- Zanamivir not recommended for patients with underlying lung disease, as may cause bronchospasm.

Influenza A & B

- Oseltamivir (treatment duration: 5 days)
  - Adult: 75 mg PO two times daily
  - Pediatric
    - 2 weeks–1 year: 3 mg/kg/dose PO two times daily
    - Age <1 year:
      - <15 kg: 30 mg PO two times daily
      - 15–23 kg: 45 mg PO two times daily
      - 24–40 kg: 60 mg PO two times daily
  - Prophylaxis: Dose for age group, but once daily for 7 days
- Zanamivir 10 mg (2 inhalations) two times daily for 5 days (age >7)
  - Prophylaxis: 10 mg (2 inhalations) once daily for 7 days (age >5)

PNEUMONIA (ADULT)

COMMUNITY-ACQUIRED
Outpatient

Common organisms: *S. pneumoniae, H. influenzae, M. pneumoniae, C. pneumoniae, Legionella spp., viruses*

Previously healthy and low-risk for drug-resistant *S. pneumoniae*

- Azithromycin 500 mg PO once daily for day 1, *THEN* 250 mg PO once daily for days 2 through 5
- Clarithromycin 500 mg PO two times daily for 7–10 days
- Doxycycline 100 mg PO two times daily for 7–10 days

Significant Comorbidities

- Levofloxacin 750 mg PO daily for 5 days
- Moxifloxacin 400 mg PO daily for 7–10 days
- Amoxicillin/clavulanate 2 g PO two times daily *PLUS*
  - Azithromycin 500 mg PO once daily for day 1, *THEN* 250 mg PO once daily for days 2 through 5 *OR*
  - Clarithromycin 500 mg PO two times daily for 7–10 days *OR*
  - Doxycycline 100 mg PO two times daily for 7–10 days

Inpatient, Non-ICU

Common organisms: As above, plus *M. catarrhalis, Klebsiella spp., S. aureus*

- Ceftriaxone 1 g IV once daily *PLUS*
  - Azithromycin 500 mg IV/PO once daily *OR*
  - Doxycycline 100 mg IV/PO two times daily
- Levofloxacin 750 mg IV/PO once daily
- Moxifloxacin 400 mg IV/PO once daily

No Pseudomonas Risk, ICU

Common organisms: As above, plus *S. pneumoniae* (drug-resistant)

- Ceftriaxone 1 g IV once daily *PLUS*
  - Azithromycin 500 mg IV once daily *OR*
  - Levofloxacin 750 mg IV once daily *OR*
  - Moxifloxacin 400 mg IV once daily
- If penicillin allergic: aztreonam 2 g IV three times daily *AND* levofloxacin 750 mg IV once daily
- If MRSA suspected, *ADD* vancomycin 15–20 mg/kg IV two times daily

Pseudomonas Risk, ICU or Non ICU

Common organisms: As above, plus *Pseudomonas spp.*

- Levofloxacin 750 mg IV once daily *PLUS*
  — Cefepime 2 g IV three times daily *OR*
  — Piperacillin/tazobactam 4.5 g IV four times daily
- Gentamicin 5–7 mg/kg IV once daily *AND* azithromycin 500 mg IV once daily *PLUS*
  — Cefepime 2 g IV three times daily *OR*
  — Piperacillin/tazobactam 4.5 g IV four times daily
- For severe β-lactam allergy
  — Gentamicin 5–7 mg/kg IV once daily *AND* levofloxacin 750 mg IV once daily *AND* aztreonam 2 g IV three times daily
- If MRSA suspected, *ADD* vancomycin 15–20 mg/kg IV two times daily

PEARLS

- If clinically suspected, consider treatment for influenza if within 48 hours of symptom onset.
- If antibiotic exposure in the last 3 months, use a different class of antibiotic.
- Pseudomonal risk factors:
  — Bronchiectasis
  — Structural lung disease (chronic bronchitis, COPD, interstitial lung disease) *AND* in prior 3 months
    • History of repeated antibiotic exposure *OR*
    • Chronic steroid use

AIDS, Considering *Pneumocystis Jiroveci* (PCP) Pneumonia

- CD4 count normal: treat as community-acquired pneumonia
- CD4 count <200 or clinical AIDS
- See *Pneumocystis Jiroveci* pneumonia (PCP) chapter (page 82).

Aspiration Pneumonia or Abscess

Common organisms: *Anaerobes*, gram-negative species

- Ampicillin/sulbactam 3 g IV four times daily
- Ceftriaxone 1 g IV once daily *AND* clindamycin 600 mg IV three times daily
- Piperacillin/tazobactam 4.5 g IV three times daily
- Imipenem/cilastatin 500 mg IV four times daily
- If penicillin-allergic: clindamycin 600 mg IV three times daily *PLUS*
  — Levofloxacin 750 mg IV once daily *OR*
  — Moxifloxacin 400 mg IV once daily

PULMONARY

59

Health Care-Associated Pneumonia (HCAP)
Hospital-Acquired Pneumonia (HAP) and Ventilator-Associated Pneumonia (VAP)

Common organisms: *S. pneumoniae, H. influenzae, S. aureus (including MRSA), E. coli, Klebsiella spp., Enterobacter spp., Proteus spp., S. marcescens, Pseudomonas spp., Acinetobacter spp., L. pneumophila*

- Choose one from Category A *AND* Category B *AND* Category C

Category A	Category B	Category C
■ Cefepime 2 g IV three times daily ■ Ceftazidime 2 g IV three times daily ■ Piperacillin/tazobactam 4.5 g IV four times daily ■ Imipenem/cilastatin 500 mg IV four times daily ■ If penicillin-allergic: aztreonam 2 g IV three times daily	■ Ciprofloxacin 400 mg IV three times daily ■ Levofloxacin 750 mg IV once daily ■ Gentamicin 5–7 mg/kg IV once daily (only for HAP) ■ Azithromycin 500 mg IV once daily	■ Vancomycin 15–20 mg/kg IV two times daily ■ Linezolid 600 mg IV two times daily

PEARLS

- Patients at risk for MDR pathogens: current hospitalization >5 days or antibiotic use within 90 days, hospitalization greater than 2 days over the past 3 months, known antibiotic resistance or family member with MDR pathogen, nursing home or long-term care facility residents, home infusion therapy, immunosuppressive disease and/or therapy, hemodialysis, IV antibiotics, wound care within 30 days.

PNEUMONIA (PEDIATRIC)

Outpatient

Common organisms: *Respiratory syncytial virus, Influenza, S. pneumoniae, H. influenzae, M. pneumoniae, C. pneumoniae, other viruses*

Presumed Bacterial Pneumonia
- Amoxicillin 45 mg/kg PO two times daily for 10 days
- Amoxicillin/clavulanate 45 mg/kg PO two times daily for 10 days
- Cefpodoxime 5 mg/kg PO two times daily
- If diagnosis of bacterial pneumonia is in doubt, **ADD** azithromycin 10 mg/kg PO once daily for day 1, **THEN** 5 mg/kg PO once daily for days 2 though 5.

Presumed Atypical Pneumonia
- Azithromycin 10 mg/kg PO once daily for day 1, **THEN** 5 mg/kg PO once daily for days 2 though 5
- Clarithromycin 7.5 mg/kg PO two times daily for 7–14 days
- Doxycycline 1–2 mg/kg PO two times daily (for children >7 years old) for 10–14 days

Inpatient

Common organisms: *S. pneumoniae, M. pneumoniae, C. pneumoniae, H. influenzae, S. aureus, M. catarrhalis, Legionella spp., E. coli, K. pneumoniae,* drug-resistant *S. aureus, S. pneumoniae, Pseudomonas spp.,* influenza, other viruses

Presumed Bacterial Pneumonia

Fully immunized with conjugate vaccines for *Haemophilus influenzae type b* and *Streptococcus pneumoniae*; local penicillin-resistance in invasive strains of pneumococcus is minimal
- Ampicillin 50 mg/kg IV four times daily
- Ceftriaxone 50 mg/kg IV two times daily
- Cefotaxime 50 mg/kg IV three times daily
- If MRSA suspected, **ADD** clindamycin 10 mg/kg IV four times daily **OR** vancomycin 15 mg/kg IV four times daily

Not Fully Immunized for *H. influenzae* type b and *S. pneumoniae*; local penicillin resistance in invasive strains of pneumococcus is significant

- Ceftriaxone 50 mg/kg IV two times daily
- Cefotaxime 50 mg/kg IV three times daily
- If penicillin allergic: levofloxacin 10 mg/kg IV/PO once daily (6 months to 5 years old: two times daily)
- If MRSA suspected, *ADD* clindamycin 10 mg/kg IV four times daily *OR* vancomycin 15 mg/kg IV four times daily

Presumed Atypical Pneumonia

- Azithromycin 10 mg/kg IV once daily for days 1 and 2, *THEN* 5 mg/kg IV once daily for days 3 though 5
- Clarithromycin 7.5 mg/kg PO two times daily for 7–14 days
- Doxycycline 1–2 mg/kg IV/PO two times daily (for children >7 years old)
- If penicillin-allergic: levofloxacin 10 mg/kg IV/PO once daily (6 months to 5 years old: two times daily)
- If diagnosis of atypical pneumonia is in doubt, *ADD* ampicillin 50 mg/kg IV four times daily

CUTANEOUS ABSCESS

Note: Incision and drainage (I&D) is the treatment of choice. Antibiotics are not generally indicated ("choosing wisely" recommendation).

Simple Cutaneous Abscess, Carbuncle, Furuncle

Common organisms: *Staphylococcus spp.* (including MSSA and CA-MRSA), *Streptococcus spp., Pseudomonas spp.* (chronic carbuncle), and *anaerobes;* usually *polymicrobial*

Overlying Cellulitis, Signs of Severe Infection (i.e., high fever), Immunocompromised Patient, Multiple Lesions, Size >5 cm
(treatment duration: 5–10 days unless otherwise noted)

- TMP/SMX (DS) 1–2 tablets (5 mg/kg) PO two times daily *AND* cephalexin 500 mg (12.5 mg/kg) PO four times daily
- Clindamycin 450–600 mg PO three times daily (10 mg/kg PO four times daily)
- Doxycycline 100 mg PO two times daily
- Vancomycin 15–20 mg/kg IV two times daily (10 mg/kg four times daily)

Hidradenitis Suppurativa

- A primary inflammatory process that may become secondarily infected.
- Clindamycin 1% topical lotion applied to affected area two times daily until resolved.
- Consider clindamycin 450 mg PO three times daily (duration based on clinical response).
- Referral to surgeon for definitive treatment.

Perianal Abscess

Common organisms: *Enterobacteriaceae, Pseudomonas spp., Bacteroides spp., Enterococcus spp.* (polymicrobial including gram negative and anaerobic coverage)

Note: Incision and draining (I&D) is the treatment of choice. Consider antibiotics post-procedure.

- Amoxicillin/clavulanate 875 mg PO two times daily for 7 days
- Metronidazole 500 mg (10 mg/kg) PO three times daily for 7 days *PLUS*
  - Ciprofloxacin 500 mg PO two times daily for 7 days *OR*
  - Levofloxacin 750 mg PO daily *OR*
  - Cephalexin 500 mg (12.5 mg/kg) PO four times daily *OR*
  - TMP/SMX (DS) 1–2 tablets (5 mg/kg) PO two times daily for 7 days

SKIN & SOFT TISSUE

Severe

- Vancomycin 15–20 mg/kg IV two times daily *PLUS*
  - Cefepime 2 g IV two times daily *AND*
  - Metronidazole 500 mg IV two times daily

If PCN-Allergic

- Metronidazole 500 mg IV three times daily *PLUS*
  - Levofloxacin 750 mg IV daily *AND*
  - Vancomycin 15-20 mg/kg IV two times daily

PEARLS

- All neuropathic ulcers should be assessed for infection and debrided of callus and necrotic tissue.
- Osteomyelitis should be considered in all cases of deep ulceration. Ulcers with evidence of infection and a positive probe-to-bone test are likely to be complicated by osteomyelitis.
- Plain radiographs may show foreign bodies, soft-tissue gas, or bony abnormalities, but the sensitivity and specificity is poor. MRI is the imaging modality of choice to rule out osteomyelitis.

PARONYCHIA

Common organisms: *Staphylococcus spp., Streptococcus spp., Candida spp., Pseudomonas spp.*

- Treatment is I&D of the abscess.
- Reserve antibiotics for associated cellulitis (see page 64).

FELON

Common organisms: *S. aureus, Streptococcus spp., Eikenella corrodens, Herpes simplex virus* (**Treatment is I&D and 7–10 days of antibiotic therapy**)

- Clindamycin 450–600 mg PO three times daily
- Cephalexin 500 mg PO four times daily
- TMP/SMX (DS) 1–2 tablets PO two times daily
- Dicloxacillin 250 mg PO four times daily
- Acyclovir 400 mg PO three times daily (if herpes suspected)

PEARLS

- Vesicles are consistent with herpetic infection (do not I&D).
- Ultrasound can be useful to define extent of abscess or identify foreign bodies.
- Consider combination therapy if infection with oral flora is suspected (amoxicillin/clavulanate).

FOLLICULITIS

Common organisms: *S. aureus, Pseudomonas spp.*

Topical Treatment

- Topical clindamycin 1% to affected area two times daily as needed
- Topical erythromycin 2% to affected area two times daily as needed
- Mupirocin 2% ointment to affected area three times daily as needed
- Chlorhexidine 2% containing antiseptic cleanser daily for 1–2 weeks

PEARLS

- Treatment for hot tub folliculitis is generally not indicated.

IMPETIGO

Common organisms: *S. aureus* (MSSA and CA-MRSA) and *Group A Streptococcus*

- Mupirocin 2% ointment two times daily for 5 days (for isolated lesions)
- Cephalexin 250 mg (6.25 mg/kg) PO four times daily for 7 days
- Amoxicillin/clavulanate 875 mg (12.5 mg/kg) PO two times daily for 7 days
- If MRSA suspected: clindamycin 300 mg PO four times daily (7 mg/kg PO three times daily) for 7 days

PEARLS

- Topical antibiotics are as effective as oral antibiotics for treating limited cases of nonbullous impetigo.
- Oral antibiotics should be used for bullous disease or when topical treatment is impractical because of the number of lesions.

MASTITIS

Common organisms: *S. aureus, Streptococcus spp.*

MRSA Not Suspected (treatment duration: 10 days)
- Cephalexin 500 mg PO four times daily
- Amoxicillin/clavulanate 875 mg PO two times daily
- Azithromycin 500 mg PO once daily for day 1, *THEN* 250 mg PO once daily for days 2 through 5

MRSA Suspected (treatment duration: 10 days)
- Clindamycin 450 mg PO three times daily
- TMP/SMX (DS) 2 tablets PO two times daily (consider strep coverage in addition)

PEARLS
- Symptomatic treatment includes warm compresses, analgesics, and increased frequency of breastfeeding/pumping.

NECROTIZING FASCIITIS
(INCLUDING FOURNIER'S GANGRENE, GAS GANGRENE)

Common organisms: *B. fragilis, Streptococcus spp., Staphylococcus spp., Enterococcus spp., E. coli, Clostridium spp.*
- Vancomycin 15–20 mg/kg IV two times daily *PLUS*
  - Piperacillin/tazobactam 4.5 g IV three times daily *OR*
  - Imipenem/cilastatin 1 g IV three times daily *OR*
  - Clindamycin 600 mg IV three times daily *AND* ciprofloxacin 400 mg IV two times daily

PEARLS
- Prompt surgical evaluation is critical.
- Gas in scrotal wall on U/S examination considered sonographic hallmark of Fournier's.
- Fournier's most common pathogens: *staphylococcus* and *pseudomonas*.
- CT best defines extent of disease, may identify source, and aids in surgical planning.
- Consider hyperbaric oxygen therapy if available.

SKIN & SOFT TISSUE

BARTHOLIN CYST/ABSCESS

Common organisms: polymicrobial, *E. coli, S. aureus, vaginal flora, N. gonorrhea, C. trachomatis, B. fragilis*

- Antimicrobial therapy is usually not indicated.
- See UTI Chapter (page 49) for treatment regimen if needed.

PEARLS

- Sitz baths assist with drainage.
- OB-GYN follow up for recurrent cases (for marsupialization) or perimenopausal patients (possible biopsy).
- Incision and drainage with Word catheter placement or gauze packing may be necessary.
- If risk factors for sexually transmitted disease exist, consider culture of the abscess, treatment for STD/STI, and testing for additional sexually transmitted diseases.

TINEA

Tinea Capitis

Common organisms: *Microsporum canis, Trichophyton spp.*

Use one topical treatment *AND* one systemic medication.

- Topical
  - Selenium sulfide 2.25% shampoo three times weekly for 2 weeks
  - Ketoconazole 2% shampoo three times weekly for 2 weeks
- Systemic
  - Fluconazole 150 mg (6 mg/kg) PO once weekly for 8 weeks
  - Griseofulvin 500 mg (10 mg/kg ultramicrosize, 20 mg/kg microsize, 20 mg/kg suspension) PO daily for 6–12 weeks
  - Itraconazole 200 mg (5 mg/kg) PO daily for 2–4 weeks

Tinea Corporis, Cruris, Pedis, or Manuum

Common organisms: *Trichophyton spp., Epidermophyton floccosum*

- Isolated or mild/moderate severity
  - Topical clotrimazole or ketoconazole 2 times daily for at least 4 weeks (or for 1 week after lesions have healed)

- Severe, bullous, or extensive disease
  - Fluconazole 150 mg (6 mg/kg) PO once weekly for 2–3 weeks
  - Itraconazole 200 mg (5 mg/kg) PO daily (two times daily for pedis/manuum) for 1 week
  - Griseofulvin 500–1000 mg (10 mg/kg ultramicrosize, 20 mg/kg microsize) PO daily for 2–4 weeks

Tinea Versicolor (Pityriasis Versicolor)

Common organisms: *Malassezia furfur, Pityrosporum orbiculare*

- Topical
  - Selenium sulfide 2.5% lotion, apply for 10 minutes on skin daily for 1–4 weeks; or one overnight application
  - Ketoconazole 2% cream once daily for 10–21 days
  - Zinc pyrithione 1% shampoo, apply for 10 minutes on skin daily for 1–4 weeks
- Systemic
  - Fluconazole 400 mg PO single dose
  - Itraconazole 400 mg (5 mg/kg) PO once daily for 3–7 days

PEARLS

- Systemic antifungals are associated with cases of fulminant hepatic failure. Baseline liver function tests are recommended prior to therapy. Follow-up care and ongoing monitoring of therapy are required.
- Systemic antifungals are associated with Stevens-Johnson Syndrome and drug-drug interactions through the P-450 system.
- Systemic antifungals are typically not approved for pediatric use, though documented use has indicated similar safety and efficacy as for adults.
- Itraconazole is associated with heart failure and arrhythmias have resulted from drug-drug interactions. Not recommended for patients with ventricular dysfunction or CHF.
- Griseofulvin may decrease the efficacy of oral contraceptives.
- In cases of kerion formation, oral steroids may help reduce the risk of permanent hair loss.

VARICELLA (CHICKEN POX) OR ZOSTER (SHINGLES)

Children
- Immunocompetent and less than age 12
  - No treatment
- At risk for complicated disease (age >12, cardiopulmonary disease, chronic steroid therapy, etc.)
  - Acyclovir 20 mg/kg PO four times daily for 5 days
- Immunocompromised
  - Acyclovir 10 mg/kg IV three times daily for 7 days

Adults
- Immunocompetent
  - Acyclovir 800 mg PO four times daily for 5 days (five times daily for zoster)
  - Valacyclovir 1000 mg PO three times daily for 7–14 days
  - Famciclovir 500 mg PO three times daily for 14 days
- Immunocompromised
  - Acyclovir 10 mg/kg IV three times daily for 7 days

PEARLS
- Herpes ophthalmicus — consult ophthalmology.
- Consider admission of pregnant patients with varicella.
- Complications include encephalitis, pneumonia, and hepatitis.
- Consider steroids in adults with zoster.
- Treatment should begin within 24 hours of the varicella rash, or 72 hours from zoster symptom onset.
- Acyclovir dosing is based on *ideal* body weight.

SKIN & SOFT TISSUE

ANTHRAX

In any case of suspected bioterrorism, contact your local health department and the CDC Emergency Response Hotline at 770-488-7100. Anthrax is a reportable disease and all cases should be reported to the local or state health department. These regimens are in the case of a bioterrorism-related exposure. Naturally occurring anthrax, though uncommon, may be treated with less aggressive regimens such as penicillin V 500 mg PO four times daily for 7-10 days.

Common organism: *Bacillus anthracis*

Treatment: Adult
Post-Exposure Prophylaxis (treatment duration: 60 days)
- Anthrax vaccine on days 0, 14, and 28 *PLUS*
  - Ciprofloxacin 500 mg PO two times daily *OR*
  - Doxycycline 100 mg PO two times daily

Cutaneous Anthrax *without* Signs of Toxicity (treatment duration: 60 days)
- Ciprofloxacin 500 mg PO two times daily
- Doxycycline 100 mg PO two times daily

Inhalational, Intestinal, or Cutaneous Disease *with* Signs of Toxicity (treatment duration: 60 days)
- Ciprofloxacin 400 mg IV two times daily (preferred agent) *OR*
- Doxycycline 100 mg IV two times daily (only in patients with a major contraindication to ciprofloxacin) *AND* clindamycin 900 mg IV three times daily *PLUS OR MINUS* third agent
- At least one of the agents should have good CNS penetration and in vitro activity against *B. anthracis* (meropenem, imipenem/cilastatin, rifampin, vancomycin, penicillin, or ampicillin).

Treatment: Pediatrics
Post-Exposure Prophylaxis (treatment duration: 60 days)
- Ciprofloxacin 15 mg/kg PO (max 500 mg/dose) two times daily
- Doxycycline 2.2 mg/kg PO (max 100 mg/dose) two times daily

Cutaneous Anthrax *without* Signs of Toxicity (treatment duration: 60 days)
- Ciprofloxacin 10–15 mg/kg PO (max 500 mg/dose) two times daily

Inhalational, Intestinal, or Cutaneous Disease *with* Signs of Toxicity

- Ciprofloxacin 10–15 mg/kg IV two times daily (max 400 mg/dose) {first-line agent} *OR*
- Doxycycline 2.2 mg/kg IV (max 100 mg) two times daily (only in patients with a major contraindication to ciprofloxacin) *AND* clindamycin 7.5 mg/kg IV four times daily *PLUS OR MINUS* third agent
- At least one of the agents should have good CNS penetration and in-vitro activity against *B. anthracis* (meropenem, imipenem/cilastin, rifampin, vancomycin, penicillin, or ampicillin).

PEARLS

- There is no human-to-human transmission, therefore isolation not required.
- Inhalational
  - Prodrome period: begins as an influenza-like syndrome for 2–3 days with prominent symptoms of cough and chest discomfort to help distinguish from flu.
  - Acute phase: sudden onset of hypoxia, dyspnea, shock, signs of hemorrhagic mediastinitis, hemorrhagic meningitis.
  - Gastrointestinal and oropharyngeal anthrax should be treated as inhalational.
- Cutaneous
  - Non-tender skin lesion with surrounding edema and lymphadenopathy
  - Evolves from papule to vesicle to burst vesicle with central black eschar over the course of a week.

In any case of suspected bioterrorism, contact your local health department and the CDC Emergency Response Hotline at 770-488-7100.

Common organism: *Clostridium spp.*

Foodborne Botulism

- Equine serum botulism antitoxin (for patients greater than 1 year of age)
- Skin test for sensitivity prior to administering one vial of antitoxin. Only 1 vial is necessary as circulating antitoxins only have a half life of 5–8 days.
- For antitoxin, contact local and state health departments. If not available, contact the Centers for Disease Control and Prevention at 770-488-7100.

Infant Botulism

- Only available through California Dept. of Health, Infant Botulism Program at 510-231-7600.

Inhalational Botulism

- For suspected inhalation botulism, immediately contact the Centers for Disease Control.
- Same treatment as foodborne botulism (see above).
- Inhalational botulism does not occur naturally; suspect bioterrorism.

Wound Botulism

- See Gas Gangrene chapter (page 69).

PEARLS

- Adult dx: (1) symmetric, descending flaccid paralysis with bulbar palsies (4D's: **d**iplopia, **d**ysarthria, **d**ysphonia, **d**ysphagia), (2) afebrile patient, (3) clear sensorium, (4) no sensory deficits except blurred vision (consider other dx if sensory deficit).
- Infant dx: Constipation often first, but can be overlooked; most often present with poor feeding, ptosis, lethargy, and hypotonia.
- No human-to-human transmission, therefore isolation not required.
- Foodborne botulism diagnosis is obtained by serum assay for toxin.
- Infant botulism diagnosis is obtained by direct toxin analysis and culture of stool for organism.
- Antibiotics are not routinely required for foodborne, inhalational, or infant botulism.

In any case of suspected bioterrorism, contact your local health department and the CDC Emergency Response Hotline at 770-488-7100.

Post-Exposure Prophylaxis

- Vaccinia vaccine (within 3 days of exposure)
- To obtain vaccinia vaccine, contact your State Health Department or the CDC.

Active Disease

- Vaccination within 3 days can prevent or reduce severity of disease.
- Vaccination within 7 days may modify disease course.
- Provide adequate fluid intake, pain and fever relief, and possible antibiotics for bacterial superinfection from open lesions.

Vaccine Complications

- If directly exposed to smallpox, there are no contraindications for post-exposure vaccination in an emergent setting.
- For routine vaccination, contraindications include patients at high risk for adverse events: pregnant, eczema, cardiac disease, or immunosuppressed, as well as those patients living in the same household as high-risk patients.
- Patients allergic to polymyxin, tetracycline, streptomycin, or neomycin should be excluded from routine vaccination.
- Investigational agents are available through the CDC; contact the Clinical Information Line at 877-554-4625.

PEARLS

- Follow CDC guidelines for post-vaccination care.
- Prodromal illness may include fever (101–104°) and malaise, followed by centrifugal maculopapular rash on skin (including palms, soles, and mucosa).
- All lesions on a given part of the body are in the same stage of development.
- Commonly confused with varicella (chickenpox), which has lesions that are centripetal (excluding palms and soles) and in different stages of development.
- Isolation precautions:
  - Airborne and contact transmissibility
  - Isolation in negative pressure
  - Level D personal protective equipment with N95 respirator

BIOTERRORISM

TULAREMIA

In any case of suspected bioterrorism, contact your local health department and the CDC Emergency Response Hotline at 770-488-7100.

Common organism: *Francisella tularensis,* a gram-negative coccobacillus

Post-Exposure Prophylaxis or Mass Casualty, Adult
- Doxycycline 100 mg PO two times daily for 14–21 days
- Ciprofloxacin 500 mg PO two times daily for 10 days

Active Disease or Contained Casualty Preferred (treatment duration: 10 days)
- Streptomycin 1 g (15 mg/kg) IM two times daily
- Gentamicin 5 mg/kg IV/IM once daily (2.5 mg/kg IV/IM three times daily)

Alternatives
- Ciprofloxacin 400 mg (15 mg/kg, max daily dose 1g) IV two times daily for 10 days
- Doxycycline 100 mg (2.2 mg/kg) IV two times daily for 14–21 days
- Chloramphenicol 15 mg/kg (15 mg/kg, max daily dose 4g) IV four times daily for 14–21 days

PEARLS
- No human-to-human transmission, thus no isolation required.
- *Pulmonary:* Flu-like symptoms, nonproductive cough, and respiratory distress
- *Typhoidal:* Fever, headache, substernal discomfort, abdominal pain, cough and weight loss, nausea, vomiting, and diarrhea
- *Ulceroglandular:* Local papule evolving to an ulcer, regional lymphadenopathy, fevers, chills, headache, and malaise
- For suspected pediatric exposure, immunocompromised patients or exposure in pregnancy, consult infectious disease.
- Vaccine is currently under review by the FDA, but is only available in the U.S. for laboratories.

In any case of suspected bioterrorism, contact your health department and the CDC Emergency Response Hotline at 770-488-7100.

Common organism: *Yersinia pestis*

Post-Exposure Prophylaxis (treatment duration: 7 days)

- Doxycycline 100 mg (2.2 mg/kg, max 100 mg/dose) PO two times daily
- Ciprofloxacin 500 mg (20 mg/kg) PO two times daily
- Chloramphenicol 25 mg/kg PO (max 1g/dose) four times daily (age >2, resistant strains exist)

Active Disease (treatment duration: 10 days)

- Gentamicin 5 mg/kg IV/IM once daily (2.5 mg/kg IV three times daily)
- Ciprofloxacin 500 mg (20 mg/kg) PO two times daily
- Ciprofloxacin 400 mg (15 mg/kg, max 500 mg/dose) IV two times daily
- Doxycycline 200 mg PO/IV once daily (2.2 mg/kg IV, max 100 mg/dose two times daily)
- Chloramphenicol 500 mg (25 mg/kg, max 1g/dose) IV four times daily (age >2, resistant strains exist)
- Streptomycin 1 g (15 mg/kg, max 1g/dose) IM two times daily (resistant strains exist)

PEARLS

- These regimens are effective for wild-type variants of *Yersinia pestis*; there have been reports of antibiotic-resistant strains.
- *Pneumonic:* Rapidly progressive flu-like illness with bloody sputum followed by hypoxia, shock, coagulopathy, respiratory failure
- *Bubonic:* Tender, non-fluctuant, swollen lymph nodes (buboes) in region of skin inoculation
- *Septicemic:* Bubonic plague followed by shock, DIC, and coma; acral gangrene ("black death")
- Isolation precautions:
  - Respiratory transmissibility in pneumonic form
  - Contact transmissibility in bubonic form
  - Isolation in negative pressure
  - Level D personal protective equipment with N95 respirator

ANIMAL/HUMAN BITE WOUNDS

Cat and Dog Bites, Outpatient Therapy

Common organisms: *Pasteurella spp., Streptococcus spp., Staphylococcus spp., Capnocytophaga canimorsus* (dog)
(Treatment duration: 5–7 days)

- Amoxicillin/clavulanate 875 mg (25 mg/kg) PO two times daily
- Doxycycline 100 mg PO two times daily
- Clindamycin 450 mg (5 mg/kg) PO three times daily **PLUS**
  - Ciprofloxacin 500 mg PO two times daily **OR**
  - TMP/SMX (DS) 1–2 tablets (5 mg/kg) PO two times daily
- PCN allergic pregnant women: azithromycin 250–500 mg PO once daily
  - (variable activity against *Pasteurella spp* and *Fusobacteria*)

Human Bites, Outpatient Therapy

Common organisms: *Viridans group streptococci, Bacteroides spp.,* Coagulase-negative staphylococci, *Corynebacterium spp., S. aureus, Eikenella corrodens, Fusobacterium spp., Peptostreptococcus spp.*

- Amoxicillin/clavulanate 875 mg (25 mg/kg) PO two times daily
- Metronidazole 500 mg PO three times daily **AND** ciprofloxacin 500–750 mg PO two times daily
- Moxifloxacin 400 mg PO once daily

Mammalian Bites, Inpatient Therapy

- Ampicillin/sulbactam 3 g IV (50 mg/kg IV) four times daily
- Ceftriaxone 1 g IV (50 mg/kg IV) once daily **AND** metronidazole 500 mg IV three times daily (7.5 mg/kg IV four times daily)
- Clindamycin 600 mg IV three times daily (7.5 mg/kg IV four times daily) **PLUS**
  - TMP/SMX 5 mg/kg IV two times daily **OR**
  - Ciprofloxacin 400 mg IV two times daily
- Cefoxitin 1 g IV three times daily (25 mg/kg IV four times daily)
- Pipericillin/tazobactam 4.5 g IV (80 mg/kg IV) three times daily

PEARLS

- For non-human animal bites without signs of infection, no evidence of benefit for antibiotic prophylaxis except in bites to the hand.
- Length of treatment
  - Prophylaxis 3–5 days
  - Active infection 5–7 days

78

- Obtain radiographs for hand injuries.
- Do not close puncture wounds.
- Consider rabies prophylaxis if high-risk; and tetanus prophylaxis if not up to date.

RABIES

Post-Exposure Prophylaxis, *without* Prior Vaccination
- Rabies immune globulin (RIG) 20 IU/kg (as much at wound site as possible) *AND* 1 ml deltoid IM on days 0, 3, 7, 14 of rabies vaccine

Note: Immune globulin and vaccine must be given at separate sites.

Post-Exposure Prophylaxis, *with* Prior Vaccination and Documented Antibody Response to Prior Vaccination
- 1 ml deltoid IM on days 0 and 3 of rabies vaccine

PEARLS
- Pregnancy is not a contraindication to therapy.
- Wound should be extensively cleaned with water or dilute water povidone-iodine solution.
- Administer tetanus prophylaxis if not up to date.
- Saliva is the only body fluid of an infected mammal that transmits disease.
- Domestic mammals (e.g., dogs, cats, ferrets): if the animal can be observed for 10 days and is asymptomatic, treatment is not necessary.
- Wild carnivores (e.g., skunks, raccoons, foxes, coyotes): consider rabid and begin therapy
- Bat exposure: post-exposure prophylaxis should be administered for both bite and non-bite exposures.
- Livestock, rodents (e.g., hamsters, rats, mice, gerbils, squirrels, chipmunks, rabbits): rarely carry the disease, and treatment usually not necessary.

ENVIRONMENTAL
EXPOSURES

TETANUS

Active Disease

■ Administer immunoglobulin prior to surgical debridement.
  — Human antitetanus immune globulin (TIG) 3000–6000 units IM with partial administration around identified wounds **PLUS**
    • Metronidazole 500 mg PO/IV (7.5 mg/kg PO/IV) four times daily **OR**
    • PCN G 2–4 million units (50,000 units/kg) IV four times daily
  — Administer Tdap vaccination in opposite extremity from TIG.

Prophylaxis

■ If it has been more than 5 years since patient's last booster in tetanus-prone wound or greater than 10 years in any wound:
  — Tetanus/diphtheria/acellular pertussis (Tdap) vaccine 0.5 ml IM
■ If patient has received <3 doses of primary vaccination series or status is unknown **AND** wound is tetanus-prone:
  — Human tetanus immune globulin (TIG) 250 units IM **AND**
  — Tetanus/diphtheria/acellular pertussis (Tdap) vaccine 0.5 ml IM
■ Administer Tdap vaccination in opposite extremity from TIG.

PEARLS

■ Tetanus is a clinical diagnosis; suspect if history of tetanus-prone injury and inadequate immunization. No definitive laboratory test exists.
■ Wide debridement of wound in active disease is a critical aspect of therapy to prevent further germination of spores.
■ Primary treatments are muscle relaxation (first-line benzodiazepines, second-line neuromuscular blocking agents) and airway management.
■ Incubation period can be 24 hours to several months (average 8 days); patients may not present with wound.
■ Usually shorter incubation periods are associated with increased disease severity and mortality.
■ High-risk patients for inadequate vaccination include IVDU, immigrants, rural patients, and the elderly.

CYTOMEGALOVIRUS (CMV)

Retinitis
Preferred Treatment
Vision-Threatening
- Intraocular ganciclovir implant in consultation with ophthalmologist **AND** valganciclovir 900 mg PO two times daily for 14 days, **THEN** 900 mg PO once daily for 7 days

Alternate Treatment
- Ganciclovir 5 mg/kg IV two times daily

Esophagitis or Colitis
- Ganciclovir 5 mg/kg IV two times daily for 21–28 days until symptom resolution
- Foscarnet 90 mg/kg IV two times daily for 21–28 days until symptom resolution

Pneumonia
- Ganciclovir 5 mg/kg IV two times daily for 3 weeks

CMV Neurologic Disease
- Ganciclovir 5 mg/kg IV two times daily for 21 days, **THEN** 5 mg/kg IV daily **AND** foscarnet 90 mg/kg IV two times daily for 21 days, **THEN** 90–120 mg/kg IV once daily

CRYPTOCOCCUS NEOFORMANS

Pulmonary (Non-AIDS) (treatment duration: 6-12 months)
- Fluconazole 400 mg PO/IV once daily
- Itraconazole 200 mg PO two times daily
- Voriconazole 200 mg PO two times daily
- Posaconazole 400 mg PO two times daily

Pulmonary (AIDS)
- Fluconazole 400 mg PO once daily for 6–12 months

Meningitis
- Amphotericin B deoxycholate 0.7–1 mg/kg IV once daily **AND** flucytosine 25 mg/kg PO four times daily for 4 weeks **THEN** fluconazole 400 mg PO daily for 8 weeks

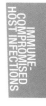

IMMUNE-COMPROMISED HOST INFECTIONS

PEARLS

- Amphotericin B deoxycholate associated with drug fevers, rigors, renal insufficiency, electrolyte disturbances and anemia.
- Consider fluids, acetaminophen, and diphenhydramine at time of infusion of amphotericin B to decrease drug infusion reactions and renal insufficiency.
- Repeated LP may be therapeutic for increased ICP.

PNEUMOCYSTIS JIROVECI PNEUMONIA (PCP)

Mild (treatment duration: 21 days)

- TMP/SMX (DS) 2 tablets PO three times daily
- Dapsone 100 mg PO once daily *AND* TMP 5 mg/kg PO three times daily
- Atovaquone 750 mg PO two times daily
- Primaquine 30 mg PO once daily *AND* clindamycin 450 mg PO three times daily

Moderate/Severe (treatment duration: 21 days)

- TMP/SMX 5 mg/kg IV three-four times daily
- Primaquine 30 mg PO once daily *AND* clindamycin 900 mg IV three times daily
- Pentamidine 4 mg/kg IV once daily over 60 minutes

Pregnant

- TMP/SMX 5 mg/kg IV three-four times daily *AND* folic acid 4 mg IV/PO once daily

PEARLS

- Corticosteroids are indicated for PaO_2 <70mm/hg or A-a gradient >35 mm/hg.
- Prednisone 40 mg two times daily for 5 days, *THEN* taper over 2 weeks.
- Dapsone may cause methemoglobinemia.

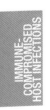

IMMUNE-
COMPROMISED
HOST INFECTIONS

TOXOPLASMOSIS

Common organism: *Toxoplasmosis gondii*

- TMP/SMX 5 mg/kg IV/PO two times daily
- Pyrimethamine 200 mg PO once, **THEN** 50–75 mg PO once daily **AND** leucovorin 10–25 mg PO once daily **PLUS**
  - Sulfadiazine 1000–1500 mg PO four times daily **OR**
  - Clindamycin 600 mg PO/IV four times daily **OR**
  - Azithromycin 1200 mg PO once daily **OR**
  - Atovaquone 1500 mg PO two times daily

PEARLS

- Patients who are immunocompetent and not pregnant usually do not require treatment unless their symptoms are severe or prolonged.
- Fatal complications include encephalitis, pneumonitis, chorioretinitis, and myocarditis.

FEBRILE NEUTROPENIA

Common organisms: *Staphylococcus spp., Streptococcus spp., Enterococcus spp., Corynebacterium spp., E. coli, Klebsiella spp., Pseudomonas spp.*

Low-Risk Outpatient

- Ciprofloxacin 750 mg PO two times daily **AND** amoxicillin/clavulanate 875 mg PO two times daily
- Levofloxacin 750 mg PO once daily

Inpatient

- Piperacillin/tazobactam 4.5 g IV four times daily
- Cefepime 2 g IV three times daily
- Imipenem/cilastatin 500 mg IV four times daily

Criteria for Including Vancomycin or Linezolid

- Catheter-related infection, PNA, cellulitis or other soft-tissue infection
- Known colonization with MRSA or multidrug-resistant *Streptococcus*
- Cultures showing gram-positive organisms with unknown susceptibility
- Hypotension/shock

Penicillin-Allergic Patient

- Ciprofloxacin 400 mg IV three times daily *AND* clindamycin 600 mg IV three times daily
- Aztreonam 2 g IV three times daily *AND* vancomycin 15–20 mg/kg IV two times daily

PEARLS

- Fever is defined as a single oral temperature of $\geq 38.3°C$, or a temperature $\geq 38.0°C$ sustained for 1 hour.
- Neutropenia is defined as ANC (absolute neutrophil count) <500 cells/mm^3, or when a drop to this level is anticipated in the next 48 hours.
- ANC <100 neutrophils/mm^3 is considered profound neutropenia and signifies higher risk.
- Antifungal therapy is not indicated in the ED, unless there is a known fungal infection.
- Antiviral therapy is generally not recommended for empiric therapy. In influenza outbreak or exposure, flu-like symptoms should prompt treatment with neuraminidase inhibitors.
- Local hospital resistance patterns should also guide antibiotic selection.
- Infrequently, a low-risk patient might be discharged from the ED on oral treatment. Determination of the patient's low-risk status and selection of therapy should be done in consultation with the patient's oncologist.
- Low-risk criteria: absolute neutrophil count ≥ 100 cells/mm^3, normal CXR, duration of neutropenia <7 days, no comorbidities, mild or no physical symptoms, cancer in remission, no evidence of fungal infection, no evidence of a catheter-site infection

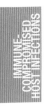

IMMUNE-
COMPROMISED
HOST INFECTIONS

HIV AND HEPATITIS

Evaluate the Exposed Person and the Source

- Wash wounds and skin with soap and water. Flush mucous membranes with water.
- Determine HCV, HBV and HIV status of source. Perform rapid HIV test, if possible.
- Assess immune status of exposed person for HBV infection (i.e., by history of hepatitis B vaccination and vaccine response). Vaccine response should be tested if not previously determined (Anti-HBs).
- Consider baseline labs per local PEP protocol.
- Note that feces, sweat, saliva, vomitus, and urine are NOT considered infectious bodily fluids.

Provide Information to the Exposed Person

- Risk of developing serologic evidence of HBV from needlestick exposure is 23–37% if blood source is HBsAg+ and HBeAg- (if HBeAg+, 37–62%).
- Multiple doses of HBIG, combined with the HBV vaccine series given within 1 week of exposure, confer greater than 75% protection from a percutaneous injury with exposure to HBsAg+ blood.
- Probability of transmission of HCV from HCV+ source via needlestick is 1.8%.
- Probability of transmission of HIV from a single exposure:
  — Percutaneous exposure (needlestick): 0.3%
  — Mucous membrane exposure: 0.09%
  — Injury with a hollow-bore needle and high viral load place exposed person at higher risk.

Give PEP for Exposure Posing Risk of Infectious Transmission

- HBV: See below
- HIV: See page 87
- Initiate PEP as soon as possible, preferably *within 2 hours of exposure.*
- Offer pregnancy testing to all women of child-bearing age.
- Treatment is presumed ineffective if started more than 72 hours after the exposure for HIV, and more than 7 days after exposure for HBV.

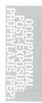

OCCUPATIONAL
POST-EXPOSURE
PROPHYLAXIS (PEP)

Hepatitis B Virus

Treatment depends on the previous vaccination history and immunity of the patient, as well as the HBV status of the source. If HBV status of source is unobtainable, estimate risk of transmission based on epidemiologic factors such as local prevalence.

Recommended Post-Exposure Prophylaxis for Exposure to Hepatitis B Virus

	Source HBsAg (+)	Source HBsAg (–)	Source unknown or not available for testing
Unvaccinated	HBIG x 1 and initiate HBV vaccine series*	Initiate HBV vaccine series	Initiate HBV vaccine series
Previously vaccinated, responder (anti-HBs >10mIU/mL)	No treatment	No treatment	No treatment
Previously vaccinated, one series, non-responder (anti-HBs <10mIU/mL)	HBIG x 1 and initiate revaccination, **OR** HBIG x 2 (now and in one month)*	No treatment	If known high-risk source, treat as if source were HBsAg (+)
Previously vaccinated, two series, non-responder (anti-HBs<10mIU/ml)	HBIG x 2	No treatment	If known high-risk source, treat as if source were HBsAg (+)

*Administer at two separate injection sites.

Treatment Dosing

- HBIG 0.06 mL/kg IM
- Vaccination series: HBV vaccine (Engerix–B 20 mcg or Recombivax HB 10 mcg IM). Repeat in 1 month, and again in 6 months.
- Pregnancy or lactation is not a contraindication to vaccination.

Hepatitis C Virus

No regimen proven beneficial for prophylaxis. For known exposures to hepatitis C, perform baseline anti-HCV, HCV RNA and ALT on exposed person. Perform follow-up testing with HCV RNA by PCR in 4-6 weeks after exposure and Anti-HCV, HCV RNA and ALT 4-6 months after exposure. If positive, refer to HCV specialist for treatment.

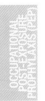

HIV

HIV PEP is time-sensitive and should be given as soon as possible. PEP should be given without waiting for source testing unless the results of a rapid test will be available within two hours. PEP is generally not warranted for unknown exposures, but should be considered if exposure source has HIV risk factors.

Recommended HIV Post-Exposure Prophylaxis

Three-drug regimens are now recommended for all HIV exposures. PEP is given for 28 days, but may be discontinued if source person testing is negative for HIV.

Preferred Three-Drug Regimen for HIV PEP

- Raltegravir 400 mg two times daily *AND*
  - Tenofovir DF 300 mg daily *AND* emtricitabine 200 mg daily (combination available as Truvada)
  - If CrCl is 30-49 ml/min, then Truvada dosing becomes every other day.
- Alternative regimens may be available with expert consultation.
- Test CBC, renal and hepatic function at baseline and two weeks after starting PEP regimen.

Resources for Consultation

- PEPline: 888-448-4911 or www.nccc.ucsf.edu/about_nccc/pepline
- HIV Antiretroviral Pregnancy Registry: 800-258-4263 or www.apregistry.com
- HIV/AIDS Treatment Information Service at www.aidsinfo.nih.gov
- Database of antiretroviral drug interactions available at www.chi.ucsf.edu

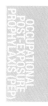
OCCUPATIONAL POST-EXPOSURE PROPHYLAXIS (PEP)

LICE — HEAD/BODY/PUBIC

OTC

- Permethrin 1% lotion — shampoo and towel-dry hair, saturate scalp with lotion, wash off after 10 minutes, *THEN* repeat in 10 days (>2 months old)
- Pyrethrin lotion — apply to affected areas, wash off after 10 minutes, *THEN* repeat in 7 days

Rx

- Spinosad 0.9% topical suspension — apply to dry scalp and hair, wash off after 10 minutes; may repeat in 7 days (>4 years old)
- Malathion 0.5% lotion — apply to affected areas, wash off after 8–12 hours; may repeat in 7 days (>6 years old)
- Benzyl alcohol 5% lotion — apply to dry hair, wash off after 10 minutes, *THEN* repeat in 7 days (>6 months old)
- Ivermectin 0.5% lotion — apply to dry hair, wash off after 10 minutes (>6 months old)
- Permethrin 5% cream — for pediculosis corporis with nits on body hair, apply to entire body, wash off after 8–10 hours
- Ivermectin — consider for patients who fail topical treatment (3 mg tablets)
  - 400 mcg/kg (pediculosis capitis) PO once on day 1, *THEN* repeat in 7 days
  - 200 mcg/kg (pediculosis corporis) PO once on day 1, *THEN* repeat in 7 days and 14 days
  - 250 mcg/kg (pediculosis pubis) PO once on day 1, *THEN* repeat in 7 days

PEARLS

- Treat close contacts.
- For eyelash infestation, apply ophthalmic-grade petroleum jelly two times daily for 10 days.
- Consider evaluation for other STDs in patients with pediculosis pubis, abstain from sexual contact until infestation clears.
- For children <2 years old, wet combing is a reasonable alternative to medical therapy.
- Children may return to school after first application of topical insecticide.
- Wash off topical medications with warm water.
- Wash clothing and bedding in hot water.
- Majority of treatments to be used in conjunction with nit combing.

PINWORMS

Common organism: *Enterobius vermicularis*

- Mebendazole 100 mg PO once, **THEN** repeat in 2 weeks
- Albendazole 400 mg PO once (100 mg if less than 2 years old), **THEN** repeat in 2 weeks
- Alternative therapy (OTC): pyrantel pamoate (Pin-X) 11 mg/kg PO once (maximum dose 1 g), **THEN** repeat every 2 weeks x 2

PEARLS

- Often asymptomatic, but may present with nocturnal perianal pruritus, abdominal pain, nausea or vomiting.
- Scotch tape applied to the perianal area can be examined microscopically for eggs.
- Consider treatment of all household contacts.
- During pregnancy, pyrantel pamoate is recommended.

SCABIES/MITES

- Permethrin 5% cream apply to entire body, wash off after 8–14 hours, **THEN** repeat in 1 week (>2 months old)
- Ivermectin 200 mcg/kg PO once, **THEN** repeat in 2 weeks (do not use in pregnant/lactating women or in peds <15 kg)
- Alternative if above not tolerated or ineffective:
  — Crotamiton 10% lotion apply daily for 2 days (apply after bathing)

PEARLS

- Wash clothing and bedding in hot water; dry clean or place in airtight bag for 72 hours.
- Treat all close contacts.

Diagnostic Criteria for Sepsis
Infection, documented or suspected, and some of the following:

- Temp >38.3°C or <36°C
- HR >90 bpm, or >two SD above the normal value for age
- Tachypnea
- WBC >12,000/uL or <4000/uL, or >10% immature forms
- Altered mental status
- Significant edema or positive fluid balance (>20 ml/kg over 24 hours)
- Hyperglycemia (plasma glucose >140 mg/dL or 7.7 mmol/L) in the absence of diabetes
- Plasma C-reactive protein more than two SD above the normal value
- Plasma procalcitonin more than two SD above the normal value
- Arterial hypotension (SBP <90 mmHg, MAP <70 mmHg, or a SBP decrease >40 mmHg in adults or less than two SD below normal for age)
- Arterial hypoxemia ($PaO_2/FiO2$ <300)
- Acute oliguria (UOP <0.5 ml/kg/hr for at least 2 hours despite adequate fluid resuscitation)
- Creatinine increase >0.5 mg/dL or 44.2 μmol/L
- Coagulation abnormalities (INR >1.5 or aPTT > 60s)
- Ileus (absent bowel sounds)
- Thrombocytopenia (platelet count <100,000/μL)
- Hyperbilirubinemia (plasma total bilirubin >4 mg/dL or 70 μmol/L)
- Hyperlactatemia (>1 mmol/L)
- Decreased capillary refill or mottling

Diagnostic Criteria for Severe Sepsis

- Sepsis-induced hypotension
- Lactate (>2 mmol/L)
- UOP <0.5 ml/kg/hr for more than two hours despite adequate fluid resuscitation
- Acute lung injury with $PaO_2/FiO2$ <250 in the absence of pneumonia as infection source
- Acute lung injury with $PaO_2/FiO2$ <200 in the presence of pneumonia as infection source
- Creatinine >2.0 mg/dL (176.8 μmol//L)
- Bilirubin >2 mg/dL (34.2 μmol/L)
- Platelet count <100,000/μL
- Coagulopathy (INR >1.5 or aPTT >60s)

Definition of Septic Shock

Sepsis-induced hypotension persisting despite adequate fluid resuscitation.

Resuscitation

- Administer broad-spectrum antibiotics (ideally within the first hour).
- Surgical source control when applicable (e.g. empyema, appendicitis)
- Intravenous (IV) fluid resuscitation (30 ml/kg bolus)

For Elevated Lactate (>4.0 mmol/L)

- Lactate assessment after each 20 ml/kg bolus
- Continued IV fluid resuscitation:
    - 20 ml/kg intravenous crystalloid bolus (0.9% normal saline)
    - Administer broad-spectrum antibiotics (ideally within the first hour)
- *Target:* lactate normalization (<2.0 mmol/L)

For Hypotension after Fluid Challenge (SBP <90, MAP <65 mmHg)

- Continued IV crystalloid resuscitation (20 ml/kg bolus) until fluid resuscitated
- Place central venous access
- Vasopressor support
    - Norepinephrine = 1st line
- Persistent hypotension
    - Vasopressin = 2nd line
    - Epinephrine infusion = 3rd line
    - Consider hydrocortisone
- Invasive monitoring
    - Consider measurement of central venous pressure (CVP): *target >8 mmHg*
    - Mixed venous oxygenation (ScvO$_2$): *target >70, <90.*
- *Target:* SBP >90, MAP >65 mmHg

PEARLS

Resuscitation

- Perform early and aggressive fluid resuscitation upon recognition of sepsis with organ dysfunction (= severe sepsis).
- Assess serial venous lactate (preferably point of care) during resuscitation targeting lactate normalization (<2 mmol/L).
- Give early central venous access and vasopressor support when sustained hypotension after IVF.
- Norepinephrine is the first-line vasopressor agent for initial support.

Empiric Antimicrobial Coverage

- Use combination therapy for neutropenic patients and for patients with risk factors for multidrug-resistant organisms, such as acinetobacter and *Pseudomonas spp.*
- Use combination therapy with a beta-lactam and either an aminoglycoside or fluoroquinolone for patients with respiratory failure and septic shock.
- Initiate antiviral therapy as early as possible for patients with severe sepsis or septic shock due to a viral etiology (e.g., oseltamivir for influenza).

NEUROCYSTICERCOSIS

Common organism: *Taenia solium* (pork tapeworm)

- Albendazole 7.5 mg/kg (400 mg/dose max) PO two times daily 8–30 days in consultation with ID
- Praziquantel 15 mg/kg PO three times daily for 15 days in consultation with ID

PEARLS

- Obtain CT head initially and consider MRI of spine if basal subarachnoid space is involved.
- Corticosteroid therapy should be administered (dexamethasone 6 mg/day or prednisone 40-60 mg/day).
- Antiparasitic therapy is NOT recommended for patients with cerebral edema or elevated ICP. Use corticosteroid therapy alone.
- Anticonvulsant therapy for CNS disease.
- Calcified cysts do not require anti-helminthic therapy.
- Obtain ophthalmology consult for ocular involvement.

EHRLICHIOSIS/ANAPLASMOSIS

Adults

- Doxycycline 100 mg PO/IV two times daily for 10 days

Children Older than Age 8

- Doxycycline 2 mg/kg PO/IV two times daily for 7–10 days

PEARLS

- Common lab findings include leukopenia, thrombocytopenia, and mildly elevated transaminases.
- Most sensitive diagnostic testing is IFA (indirect fluorescent antibody assay).
- Antibiotic therapy should not be delayed for laboratory testing in patients with suspected disease.
- Consult infectious disease for management of children and pregnant patients.
- Consider Lyme disease, Rocky Mountain spotted fever, and babesiosis in endemic areas.

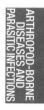

ARTHROPOD-BORNE DISEASES AND PARASITIC INFECTIONS

LYME DISEASE

Common organism: *B. burgdorferi* (tick vector: *Ixodes ricinus complex*, animal reservoir: white-footed mouse, white-tailed deer)

Prophylaxis (ALL IDSA inclusion criteria should be met: 1) *correct tick:* identified as Ixodes, 2) *correct time:* >36 hrs attached and/or engorged tick and <72 hrs since removal, 3) *correct location:* endemic area = northeast USA, some of the midwest USA, and pacific northwest.)

- Doxycycline 200 mg PO once
- If contraindication to doxycycline, follow clinically for signs of infection.

Erythema Migrans, Mild Neurologic or Cardiac Sequelae (facial nerve palsy or 1st degree AV block <300 ms) (treatment duration: 14–21 days)

- Doxycycline 100 mg (2 mg/kg) PO two times daily (*contraindicated <8 yrs or pregnant)
- Amoxicillin 500 mg (12.5 mg/kg) PO three times daily
- Cefuroxime 500 mg (15 mg/kg) PO two times daily

Serious Cardiac or Neurologic Disease: +/- Arthritis (1st degree AV block >300ms, 2nd or 3rd degree AV block, myocarditis, meningitis, CN palsies, cognitive deficits) (treatment duration: 14–28 days)

- Ceftriaxone 2 g (50–75 mg/kg) IV once daily
- Cefotaxime 2 g (75 mg/kg) IV three times daily
- Penicillin G 4M units (50,000U/kg) IV six times daily

Arthritis *without* Neurologic Sequelae (treatment duration: 28 days)

- Doxycycline 100 mg (2 mg/kg) PO two times daily
- Amoxicillin 500 mg (12.5 mg/kg) PO three times daily
- Cefuroxime 500 mg (15 mg/kg) PO two times daily

If Failure of PO Therapy, *THEN*

- Ceftriaxone 2 g (50–75 mg/kg) IV once daily

Pregnant

- **Avoid** doxycycline and clarithromycin; use alternatives as above depending on clinical presentation.
- If PCN allergic: azithromycin 500 mg (10 mg/kg) PO once daily for 7–10 days (high rate of clinical failure)

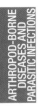

Tick Removal

- Grasp tick as close to the skin surface as possible with fine needle-nose pickups or tweezers. Do not "pop" the tick.
- Pull directly upwards away from the skin; no twisting or jerking.
- If tick mouth parts remain in skin, attempt to remove with tweezers/ superficial dissection. If in a setting without the ability to perform superficial dissection, let skin heal with mouth parts in place.
- Clean skin with iodine scrub or soap and water.

PEARLS

- Consider concomitant tick-borne diseases: babesiosis and anaplasmosis (ehrlichiosis).
- Treatment is not indicated for asymptomatic seropositive patients.
- If necessary, consider penicillin desensitization for serious cardiac or neurologic disease.
- Current treatment is identical for S.T.A.R.I. (southern tick-associated rash illness).

MALARIA

Common organisms: *P. falciparum, P. vivax, P. ovale, P. malariae*

Clinical Presentation of Uncomplicated Malaria

- Symptoms non-specific and commonly consist of fever, malaise, weakness, headache, myalgia, and chills.
- Can be confused with a viral syndrome.

P. falciparum or Species Not Identified, Chloroquine-Resistant or Unknown Resistance (all malarious regions, except those identified as chloroquine-sensitive, see PEARLS)

Adult — Any *ONE* of the Four Following Regimens

- Atovaquone/proguanil (malarone) adult tab = 250 mg atovaquone/ 100 mg proguanil
  - 4 adult tabs PO once daily for 3 days
- Artemether/lumefantrine (coartem) 1 tablet = 20 mg artemether/ 120 mg lumefantrine
  - A 3-day treatment schedule with a total of 6 oral doses is recommended for both adult and pediatric patients, based on

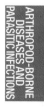

ARTHROPOD-BORNE
DISEASES AND
PARASITIC INFECTIONS

95

weight. The patient should receive the initial dose, followed by the second dose 8 hours later, *THEN* 1 dose PO two times daily for the following 2 days.

- 5–14 kg: 1 tablet per dose
- 15–24 kg: 2 tablets per dose
- 25–35kg: 3 tablets per dose
- >35 kg: 4 tablets per dose

■ Quinine sulfate 8.3 mg base/kg PO three times daily for 3 or 7 days (see PEARLS) *PLUS*
  — Doxycycline 100 mg PO two times daily for 7 days *OR*
  — Tetracycline 250 mg PO four times daily for 7 days *OR*
  — Clindamycin 20 mg base/kg/day PO divided three times daily for 7 days

■ Mefloquine (lariam) 684 mg base (750 mg salt) PO as initial dose, *THEN* 456 mg base (500 mg salt) PO given 6–12 hours after initial dose. Total dose = 1,250 mg salt

Pediatric — Any *ONE* of the Following Regimens

■ Atovaquone/proguanil (malarone)
Adult tablet = 250 mg atovaquone/100 mg proguanil
Pediatric tablet = 62.5 mg atovaquone/25 mg proguanil
  — 5–8 kg: 2 pediatric tablets PO once daily for 3 days
  — 9–10 kg: 3 pediatric tablets PO once daily for 3 days
  — 11–20 kg: 1 adult tablet PO once daily for 3 days
  — 21–30 kg: 2 adult tablets PO once daily for 3 days
  — 31–40 kg: 3 adult tablets PO once daily for 3 days
  — >40 kg: 4 adult tablets PO once daily for 3 days

■ Artemether/lumefantrine (coartem) 1 tablet = 20 mg artemether/120 mg lumefantrine
  — A 3-day treatment schedule with a total of 6 oral doses is recommended for both adult and pediatric patients, based on weight. The patient should receive the initial dose, followed by the second dose 8 hours later, *THEN* 1 dose PO two times daily for the following 2 days.
    - 5–14 kg: 1 tablet per dose
    - 15–24 kg: 2 tablets per dose
    - 25–35 kg: 3 tablets per dose
    - >35 kg: 4 tablets per dose

■ Quinine sulfate 8.3 mg base/kg (10 mg salt/kg) PO 3 times daily for 3 or 7 days (see PEARLS) *PLUS*
  — Doxycycline 2.2 mg/kg PO two times daily for 7 days (not for <8 y/o) *OR*

- — Tetracycline 6 mg/kg PO four times daily for 7 days (not for <8 y/o) **OR**
- — Clindamycin 7 mg/kg PO three times daily for 7 days (for all ages)
- Mefloquine (lariam) 13.7 mg base/kg (15 mg salt/kg) PO as initial dose, **THEN** 9.1 mg base/kg (10 mg salt/kg) PO given 6–12 hours after initial dose. Total dose = 25 mg salt/kg.

P. malariae, P. knowlesi and P. falciparum or Species Not Identified, Chloroquine-Sensitive

Adult

- Chloroquine phosphate 600 mg base (1 gram salt) PO immediately, **THEN** 300 mg base (500 mg salt) PO at 6, 24, and 48 hours for a total dose of 1,500 mg (2,500 mg salt)
- Hydroxychloroquine 620 mg base (800 mg salt) PO immediately, **THEN** 310 mg base (400 mg salt) PO at 6, 24, and 48 hours for a total dose of 1,550 mg base (2,000 mg salt)

Pediatric

- Chloroquine phosphate 10 mg base/kg PO immediately, **THEN** 5 mg base/kg PO at 6, 24, and 48 hours (total dose 25 mg base/kg)
- Hydroxychloroquine 10 mg base/kg immediately, **THEN** 5 mg/base/kg PO at 6, 24, and 48 hours (total dose of 25 mg base/kg)

P. vivax and P. ovale, Chloroquine-Sensitive (except *P. vivax* in Papua New Guinea and Indonesia, see next section)

Adult

- Chloroquine phosphate 600 mg base (1 gram salt) PO immediately, **THEN** 300 mg base (500 mg salt) PO at 6, 24 and 48 hours for a total dose 1,500 mg (2,500 mg salt) **AND** primaquine phosphate 30 mg base PO once daily for 14 days, **OR**
- Hydroxychloroquine 620 mg base (800 mg salt) PO immediately, **THEN** 310 mg base (400 mg salt) PO at 6, 24, and 48 hours for a total dose of 1,550 mg base (2,000 mg salt) **AND** primaquine phosphate 30 mg base PO once daily for 14 days

Pediatric

- Chloroquine phosphate 10 mg base/kg PO immediately, **THEN** 5 mg base/kg PO at 6, 24, and 48 hours (total dose 25 mg base/kg) **AND** primaquine phosphate 0.5 mg base/kg PO once daily for 14 days **OR**
- Hydroxychloroquine 10 mg base/kg immediately, **THEN** 5 mg/base/kg PO at 6, 24, and 48 hours (total dose of 25 mg base/kg) **AND** primaquine phosphate 0.5 mg base/kg PO once daily for 14 days

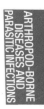

P. vivax, Chloroquine-Resistant (Papua New Guinea and Indonesia)
Adult — Any *ONE* of the three following regimens

- Quinine sulfate 542 mg base (650 mg salt) PO three times daily for 3 or 7 days (see PEARLS page 101) *PLUS*
  - Primaquine phosphate 30 mg base PO once daily for 14 days *PLUS*
    - Doxycycline 100 mg PO two times daily for 7 days *OR*
    - Tetracycline 250 mg PO four times daily for 7 days
- Atovaquone/proguanil (malarone) 4 adult tabs PO once daily for 3 days *AND* primaquine phosphate 30 mg base PO once daily for 14 days
- Mefloquine (lariam) 684 mg base (750 mg salt) PO as initial dose, *THEN* 456 mg base (500 mg salt) PO given 6–12 hours after initial dose. Total dose = 1,250 mg salt *AND* primaquine phosphate 30 mg base PO once daily for 14 days.

Pediatric — Any *ONE* of the three following regimens

- Mefloquine (lariam) 13.7 mg base/kg (15 mg salt/kg) PO as initial dose, *THEN* 9.1 mg base/kg (10 mg salt/kg) PO given 6–12 hours after initial dose
  Total dose = 25 mg salt/kg *AND* primaquine phosphate 0.5 mg base/kg PO once daily for 14 days
- Quinine sulfate 8.3 mg base/kg (10 mg salt/kg) PO 3 times daily for 3 or 7 days (see PEARLS page 101) *PLUS*
  - Primaquine phosphate 0.5 mg base/kg PO once daily for 14 days *AND*
  - Tetracycline 6 mg/kg PO four times daily for 7 days (not for <8 y/o)
- Atovaquone/proguanil (malarone)
  Adult tablet = 250 mg atovaquone/100 mg proguanil
  Pediatric tablet = 62.5 mg atovaquone/25 mg proguanil
  - 5–8 kg: 2 pediatric tablets PO once daily for 3 days
  - 9–10 kg: 3 pediatric tablets PO once daily for 3 days
  - 11–20 kg: 1 adult tablet PO once daily for 3 days
  - 21–30 kg: 2 adult tablets PO once daily for 3 days
  - 31–40 kg: 3 adult tablets PO once daily for 3 days
  - >40 kg: 4 adult tablets PO once daily for 3 days *AND* primaquine phosphate 0.5 mg base/kg PO once daily for 14 days

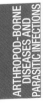

Pregnant Women
Chloroquine-Sensitive

- Chloroquine phosphate 600 mg base (1 gram salt) PO, **THEN** 300 mg base (500 mg salt) PO at 6, 24, and 48 hours. Total dose 1,500 mg (2,500 mg salt) **OR** hydroxychloroquine 620 mg base (800 mg salt) PO immediately, **THEN** 310 mg base (400 mg salt) PO at 6, 24, and 48 hours after the initial does for a total dose of 1,550 mg base (2,000 mg salt)

Chloroquine-Resistant *P. falciparum* and *P. vivax*

- Quinine sulfate 542 mg base (650 mg salt) PO three times daily for 3 or 7 days (see PEARLS) **AND** clindamycin 600 mg PO three times daily for 7 days
- Mefloquine (lariam) 684 mg base (750 mg salt) PO as initial dose, **THEN** 456 mg base (500 mg salt) PO given 6–12 hours after initial dose. Total dose = 1,250 mg salt

Clinical Presentation of Complicated (Severe) Malaria
(usually due to *P. falciparum*)

As defined by one or more of the following: Impaired consciousness/coma, renal failure, pulmonary edema, shock, jaundice, disseminated intravascular coagulation, and/or parasitemia of >5%

Adult

- Quinidine gluconate 6.25 mg base/kg (10 mg salt/kg) loading dose IV over 1–2 hrs, **THEN** 0.0125 mg base/kg/min (0.02 mg salt/kg/min) continuous infusion for at least 24 hours **PLUS**
  - Doxycycline 100 mg IV/PO two times daily for 7 days **OR**
  - Tetracycline 250 mg PO four times daily for 7 days **OR**
  - Clindamycin 10 mg/kg PO load then 5 mg/kg PO three times daily for 7 days

Pediatric

- Quinidine gluconate: 6.25 mg base/kg (10 mg salt/kg) loading dose IV over 1–2 hrs, then 0.0125 mg base/kg/min (0.02 mg salt/kg/min) continuous infusion for at least 24 hours **PLUS**
  - Clindamycin 7 mg/kg PO three times daily for 7 days
  - Doxycycline 2.2 mg/kg PO two times daily for 7 days
    - If unable to take PO: <45 kg: 2.2 mg/kg IV two times daily, for >45 kg use same dosing for adults for 7 days **OR**
  - Tetracycline 6 mg/kg PO four times daily for 7 days (not for < 8 y/o)

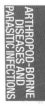

ARTHROPOD-BORNE
DISEASES AND
PARASITIC INFECTIONS

PEARLS

- Suspect in any febrile patient returning from the tropics.
- Chloroquine-sensitive areas include Haiti, Dominican Republic, Central America west of the Panama Canal, and most of the Middle East.
- For country-specific resistance patterns and country-specific species, see the CDC's website: www.cdc.gov/malaria/travelers/country_table.
- If a patient develops malaria while on chemoprophylaxis, that particular medication should not be used as part of the treatment regimen, and an alternative option should be selected.
- Call the CDC with any failure of treatment.
- Thick and thin blood smears every 12 to 24 hours for a total of 3 sets to make diagnosis; one negative smear is never enough to rule out suspected malaria.
- *Plasmodium vivax* and *P. ovale* infections require treatment with primaquine for the hypnozoites that remain dormant in the liver and can cause a relapsing infection, but not for pregnant women.
- Pediatric dosing should **NEVER** exceed adult dosing.
- Primaquine can cause hemolytic anemia in persons with G6PD deficiency.
- Mefloquine noted to cause neuropsychiatric reactions in some patients.
- Quinidine can lead to arrhythmias (QT as well as QRS prolongation), and hypotension; always administer with cardiac monitoring. It can also lead to hypoglycemia, a common side effect. Therefore, blood glucose should be monitored closely.
- Quinine treatment should continue for 7 days for infections acquired in Southeast Asia and for 3 days for infections acquired in Africa or South America.
- RBC exchange transfusion should be considered for the most severe cases such as parasite density >10%, ARDS, renal complications, or cerebral malaria.
- Pregnant women diagnosed with severe malaria should be aggressively treated with parenteral therapy; tetracycline, doxycycline and primaquine are contraindicated.
- Artemisinin resistance has been identified on some Asian isolates (Cambodia and Thailand).
- Artesunate, a new investigational drug and not FDA approved, may be used for the treatment of severe malaria in coordination with the CDC.

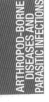

ARTHROPOD-BORNE DISEASES AND PARASITIC INFECTIONS

ROCKY MOUNTAIN SPOTTED FEVER

Common organism: *R. rickettsii*
- Doxycycline 100 mg (2.2 mg/kg), PO/IV two times daily for 5–10 days
- Pregnant/allergic: Consult infectious disease.

PEARLS
- Current recommendations are to treat for at least 3 days after the fever subsides and until evidence of clinical improvement is noted, which is typically a minimum of 5–7 days.
- Doxycycline is considered the drug of choice for children with RMSF. The risk of dental staining is minimal with one course of doxycycline.
- Consider doxycycline 200 mg IV loading dose for seriously ill patients.
- Prophylaxis following tick bite to prevent infection not recommended.

Cephalosporins

- Common reactions include: GI upset, rash, headache, dizziness, as well as elevated liver transaminases.
- Ceftriaxone should not be administered to any patient less than 28 days old as has been shown to cause increased hyperbilirubinemia and precipitation of calcium into lungs and kidneys of neonates.
- Use has also been shown to be associated with angioedema, thrombocytopenia, hemolytic anemia, hepatitis, and increased risk for superinfections.

Linezolid

- Common reactions include GI upset, headache, and fever.
- Use with caution with SSRIs, due to increased risk of serotonin syndrome.
- Use has also been associated with myelosuppression (after 2 weeks of therapy), peripheral and optic neuropathy, lactic acidosis as well as increased risk for superinfections.

Metronidazole

- Common reactions include GI upset, headache, confusion, ataxia, and metallic taste.
- To avoid disulfiram-like reaction, do not use within 72 hours of ethanol use.
- Prolonged use is associated with CNS effects (including aseptic meningitis, seizures, neuropathies) as well as increased risk for superinfections.

Nitrofurantoin

- Contraindicated when CrCl <60 ml/min.
- Useful for lower UTI only.
- Use has been known to cause hemolytic anemia; therefore, do not use in patients with G6PD deficiency, infants less than 1 month old, or pregnant patients at term (from 38–42 weeks).

Penicillins

- Common reactions include: GI upset (>10% of patients), fevers and rashes, especially in patients with mononucleosis (>50%).
- Cautions with usage, as many patients are hypersensitive
- Amoxicillin and amoxicillin/clavulanate: take with meals to decrease GI side effects

- Use has also been associated with thrombocytopenia, hemolytic anemia, and seizures (especially at high doses in patients with renal failure).

Quinolones
- Common reactions include GI upset, headaches, dizziness, and altered mental status (especially in the elderly).
- Avoid in children less than 18 years old, as may cause arthropathy in weight-bearing joints.
- Take at least 1 hour before or 2 hours after antacids, or other drug products containing calcium, iron, or zinc.
- May decrease elimination of methylxanthines (e.g., theophylline) and caffeine.
- Use has been shown to cause a lower seizure threshold (especially if given with NSAIDs), QT prolongation, hypo/hyperglycemia, hematologic toxicity.
- Black box warnings include tendonitis/tendon rupture (especially in patients taking corticosteroids, organ transplants, and >60 years old), as well as myasthenia gravis exacerbation.

Trimethoprim/Sulfamethoxazole
- Common reactions include GI upset, rash, and photosensitivity.
- Sulfonamides have a high incidence of hypersensitivity reactions.
- Patients should be advised to maintain adequate hydration due to potential transient elevation of creatinine and potassium.
- TMP/SMX is pregnancy category C in the first and second trimesters, as trimethoprim interferes with folic acid metabolism. TMP/SMX is pregnancy category D in the third trimester, and contraindicated because it can cause kernicterus.
- Do not give to patients with G6PD deficiency.
- Use has been shown to cause dose-dependent blood dyscrasias, including thrombocytopenia, megaloblastic anemia, and neutropenia.

Tetracyclines
- Common reactions include GI upset and photosensitivity.
- Do not use in children younger than 8, as stains teeth and retards bone growth.
- Contraindicated in pregnancy and lactation: pregnancy class D.
- Potentiates digoxin levels.
- Avoid antacids, dairy products, and iron within 2 hours of ingestion.
- Doxycycline taken with food to prevent GI upset outweighs the 20% decrease in absorption.

■ Take on an empty stomach, but drink a lot of water and do not take before sleep; has been shown to cause esophageal ulceration and strictures.

Vancomycin
■ May cause "red man syndrome": flushing, erythema, and pruritus, usually affecting the upper body, neck, and face.
■ May also see pains and muscle spasms in the back and chest, dyspnea, and hypotension. Decreasing the IV infusion rate is recommended.
■ This medication can be nephrotoxic and requires renal dosing.
■ Prolonged use is associated with neutropenia and increased risk for superinfections.

Warfarin and Antibiotics
■ Use antibiotics with caution in patients taking warfarin. Patient may need follow up for INR measurement within 48–72 hours.
■ The following medications
  — DECREASE the effect of warfarin: dicloxacillin, griseofulvin, nafcillin, and rifampin
  — INCREASE the effect of warfarin: azole antifungals, cephalosporins, chloramphenicol, isoniazid, macrolides, metronidazole, quinolones, sulfonamides, tigecycline

Prolonged QT and Antibiotics
■ These antimicrobials commonly prolong the QT interval: azole antifungals, macrolides, pentamidine, quinolones, trimethoprim-sulfamethoxazole

Anticonvulsants and Antibiotics
■ Multiple antibiotics interfere with the metabolism of anticonvulsants, especially phenytoin. Review potential drug interactions before prescribing new antibiotics to patients taking anticonvulsants.

G6PD Deficiency and Antibiotics
■ Avoid dapsone, mafenide cream, nalidixic acid, nitrofurantoin, primaquine, sulfacetamide, sulfamethoxazole, sulfanilamide, sulfapyridine and phenazopyridine.

Remember: All antibiotics cross the placenta.

Treatment of Urinary Tract Infections in Pregnancy
Cystitis and Asymptomatic Bacteriuria
(treatment duration: 3–7 days)

- Nitrofurantoin 100 mg PO two times daily: **Category B**
- Cefpodoxime 100 mg PO two times daily: **Category B**
- Amoxicillin 500 mg PO two times daily: **Category B**. Consider amoxicillin/clavulanate depending on resistance patterns.

Pyelonephritis Treatment in Pregnancy
(treatment duration: 10–14 days)

Mild to Moderate Disease

- Ampicillin 1–2 g IV every 6 hours *PLUS* gentamicin 1.5 g IV three times daily **Category B**
- Ceftriaxone 1 g IV once daily: **Category B**
- Cefepime 1 g IV two times daily: **Category B**
- Aztreonam 1 g IV two to three times daily: **Category B**

Severe *with* Immunocompromise *and/or* Incomplete Urinary Drainage

- Piperacillin/tazobactam 3.375 g IV four times daily: **Category B**
- Meropenam 500 mg IV three times daily: **Category B**
- Imipenem 500 mg IV four times daily: **Category B**
- Ticarcillin/clavulanate 3.1 g IV four times daily: **Category B**

Treatment of Pelvic Infections in Pregnancy
Vaginitis in Pregnancy

Bacterial Vaginosis (BV) — Always treat *symptomatic* BV in the first trimester and *all* BV beyond the first trimester. Treat *asymptomatic* BV in women at high risk for preterm labor.

- Clindamycin 900 mg three times daily *PLUS* gentamicin loading dose 2 mg/kg, followed by maintenance dose 1.5 mg/kg three times daily
- Metronidazole 500 mg PO two times daily for 7 days
- Clindamycin 300 mg PO two times daily for 7 days

Vulvovaginal candidiasis — Only topical azole therapies are recommended in pregnancy.

- Clotrimazole 1% cream 5 g intravaginally daily for 5–7 days
- Miconazole 2% cream 5 g intravaginally daily for 7 days

Trichomoniasis — Avoid intercourse until partner treated.
- Metronidazole 2 g PO once

Cervicitis and Urethritis in Pregnancy — Repeat testing 3 weeks after treatment recommended for pregnant women to confirm cure.

Gonorrhea
- Ceftriaxone 250 mg IM as a single dose
- Cefixime 400 mg PO as a single dose
- Azithromcyin 2 g PO as a single dose can be considered in women who cannot tolerate cephalosporins.

Chlamydia
- Azithromcyin 1 g PO as a single dose
- Amoxicillin 500 mg PO 3 times a day for 7 days

Pelvic Inflammatory Disease in Pregnancy

Consider admission for parenteral treatment due to risk for mother and fetus.
- Clindamycin 900 mg three times daily *PLUS* gentamicin loading dose 2 mg/kg, followed by maintenance dose 1.5 mg/kg three times daily

Antibiotics That Should Be Used with Caution or Are Contraindicated in Pregnancy
- Clarithromycin: Category C
- Quinolones: Category C
- Tetracycline/doxycycline: Category D
- Nitrofurantoin: Category B — first-line treatment during second and third trimester. Ok in first trimester if no alternative. Avoid during breastfeeding in infants with hyperbilirubinemia or G6PD deficiency; otherwise considered safe.
- Trimethoprim/sulfamethoxazole: Category C
- Gentamycin: Category C — most widely used aminoglycoside in pregnancy; reserved for resistant gram-negative infections.

CEPHALOSPORIN REFERENCE

1st Generation Cephalosporins		
Generic	**Trade**	**Route**
Cefadroxil	Duricef, Ultracef	PO
Cephalexin	Biocef, Keflex, Keftab	PO
Cephradine	Velosef	PO
Cefazolin	Ancef, Kefzol, Zolicef	IM/IV
2nd Generation Cephalosporins		
Generic	**Trade**	**Route**
Cefaclor	Ceclor	PO
Cefprozil	Cefzil	PO
Cefuroxime axetil	Ceftin	PO
Cefoxitin	Mefoxin	IV
Cefuroxime sodium	Kefurox, Zinacef	IM/IV
Cefotetan	Cefotan	IM/IV
3rd Generation Cephalosporins		
Generic	**Trade**	**Route**
Cefdinir	Omnicef	PO
Cefditoren	Spectracef	PO
Ceftibuten	Cedax	PO
Cefixime	Suprax	PO
Cefpodoxime proxetil	Vantin, Proxetil	PO
Ceftazidime	Tazicef, Tazidime, Fortaz	IV
Cefotaxime	Claforan	IV
Ceftizoxime	Cefizox	IM/IV
Cefoperazone	Cefobid	IM/IV
Ceftriaxone	Rocephin	IM/IV
4th Generation Cephalosporins		
Generic	**Trade**	**Route**
Cefepime	Maxipime	IV
5th Generation Cephalosporins		
Generic	**Trade**	**Route**
Ceftaroline	Teflaro	IV

PREGNANCY GUIDE AND METABOLISM/ EXCRETION TABLE

Antibiotic	Cost	Pregnancy Class	Lactation Safety	Metabolism/ Excretion
Abacavir	$$$$	C	U	H / R, F
Abacavir/lamivudine/ zidovudine	$$$$$	C	N	See individual medications
Acyclovir	$	B	S	O / R, F
Adefovir	$$$$$	C	U	I / R
Albendazole	$$	C	U	H / R, B
Amantadine	$	C	N	N / R
Amikacin	$$$	D	N	N / R
Ampicillin	$$	B	PS	H / R
Ampicillin/sulbactam	$$$$$	B	PS	H / R, B
Amoxicillin	$	B	S	H / R , B
Amoxicillin/clavulanate	$$$	B	PS	H / R
Amphotericin B	$$$$$	B	U	U / R
Atazanavir	$$$$$	B	N	H / F, R
Atovaquone	$$$$$	C	U	N / F, R
Azithromycin	$$	B	U	H / B, R
Aztreonam	$$$$$	B	PS	H / R, F
Caspofungin	$$$$$	C	U	H / R, F
Cefaclor	$$$	B	U	H / R
Cefadroxil	$$/$$$$	B	PS	U / R
Cefazolin	$$$	B	S	H / R
Cefepime	$$$$$	B	PS	H / R
Cefixime	$$$$$	B	U	N / R, B
Cefotaxime	$$$$$	B	PS	H / R
Cefotetan	_	B	U	N / R, B
Cefoxitin	$$$$$	B	S	N / R
Cefpodoxime/cefdinir/ cefditoren	$$$$	B	PS	G / R
Cefprozil	$$$$	B	PS	O / R
Ceftaroline	$$$$$	B	U	O / R, F
Ceftazidime	$$$$$	B	PS	N / R

Antibiotic	Cost	Pregnancy Class	Lactation Safety	Metabolism/ Excretion
Ceftibuten	$$$$	B	U	O / R
Ceftizoxime	$$$$$	B	U	N / R
Ceftriaxone	$$$$$	B	PS	O / R, F
Cefuroxime	$$$	B	PS	N / R
Cephalexin	$	B	S	N / R
Chloramphenicol	$$$$$	C	PN	H /F, B, R
Chloroquine phosphate	$$	C	PS	H / R, F
Cidofovir	$$$$$	C	U	I / R
Ciprofloxacin	$$	C	PN	H / R, F
Clarithromycin	$$$	C	U	H / R, F
Clindamycin	$	B	PN	H / R, F, B
Clotrimazole	$$$$	C	U	N/ B, F, R
Cycloserine	_	C	PS	H / R, F
Dapsone	$	C	PN	H / R
Daptomycin	$$$$$	B	U	U / R, F
Delavirdine	$$$	C	N	H / R, F
Dicloxacillin	$$	B	U	H / R, B
Didanosine	$$$$$	B	N	I / R
Doxycycline	$	D	N	H / F, R
Efavirenz	$$$$$	D	N	H / F, R
Emtricitabine	$$$$$	B	N	I / R, F
Emtricitabine/tenofovir	$$$$$	B	N	See individual medications
Enfuvirtide	$$$$$	B	N	O / U
Entecavir	$$$$$	C	U	N / R
Ertapenem	$$$$$	B	U	O / R, F
Erythromycin	$$	B	PS	H / B, R
Ethambutol	$$$$	C	PS	H / R, F
Ethionamide	$$$$$	C	U	H / R
Famciclovir	$$	B	U	H / R, F
Fluconazole	$	C (single dose), D	PS	H / R, F
Flucytosine	$$$$$	C	U	G / R, F
Fosamprenavir	$$$$$	C	N	G, H / F, R

Antibiotic	Cost	Pregnancy Class	Lactation Safety	Metabolism/Excretion
Foscarnet	$$$$$	C	U	N / R
Fosfomycin	$$	B	U	N / R, F
Ganciclovir	$$$$$	C	N	N / R
Gentamicin	$$	D	PS	N / R
Griseofulvin	$$$	C	U	H / F, R, S
Hydroxychloroquine	$$$	C	PS	H / R, B
Imipenem/cilastin	$$$$$	C	U	R / R
Indinavir	$$$$$	C	N	H / F, R
Isoniazid	$	C	PS	H / R, F
Itraconazole	$$$$$	C	U	H / R, B
Ivermectin	$	C	U	H / F, R
Ketoconazole	$$$	C	U	H / B, F, R
Lamivudine	$$$$$	C	N	I / R
Lamivudine/zidovudine	$$$$$	C	N	H, I / R
Levofloxacin	$$$$	C	PN	N / R
Linezolid	$$$$$	C	U	O / R, F
Mebendazole	$$	C	U	H / F, R
Mefloquine	$$	B	U	H / B, F
Meropenem	$$$$$	B	U	R / R
Metronidazole	$	B	U	H / R, F
Micafungin	$$$$$	C	U	H / F, R
Miconazole	$	C	U	H / F, R
Minocycline	$$$	D	PN	H / F, R
Moxifloxacin	$$$	C	PN	H / F, R
Nafcillin	$$$$$	B	PS	H / B, R
Nelfinavir	$$$$$	B	N	H / F, R
Nevirapine	$$$$$	B	N	H / R, F
Nitazoxanide	$$$	B	U	H, G, O / B, F, R
Nitrofurantoin	$$$	B	PS	I / R, B
Nystatin	$$$	C	U	N / F
Ofloxacin	$$$	C	PN	H / R, F, B
Oseltamivir	$$$	C	U	H / R, F
Oxacillin	$$$$$	B	U	H / R, B

Antibiotic	Cost	Pregnancy Class	Lactation Safety	Metabolism/ Excretion
Palivizumab	$$$$$	C	U	O / O
Paromomycin	$$$	C	PS	N / F
Penicillin	$-$$$	B	S	H / R
Pentamidine	$$$	C	N	H / R
Piperacillin/tazobactam	$$/$$$$$	B	PS	H / R, B
Praziquantel	$$$	B	PS	H / R, F
Primaquine	$	C	U	H / R
Pyrantel	$	C	U	H / F, R
Pyrazinamide	$$$$$	C	U	H / R
Pyrimethamine	$$	C	PS	H / R
Quinine	$	C	PS	H / F, R
Ribavirin	$$$$$	X	PN	H, I / R, F
Rifabutin	$$$$$	B	U	H / R, F
Rifampin	$$$$	C	PS	H / B, R
Rifapentine	$$$$	C	U	H / F, R
Rimantadine	$$	C	PN	H / R
Ritonavir	$$$$$	B	N	H / F, R
Saquinavir	$$$$$	B	N	H / F, R
Stavudine	$$$$$	C	N	I / R, F
Streptomycin	$$$$$	D	PS	N / R
Tenofovir	$$$$$	B	U	I / R
Terbinafine	$	B	U	H / R, F
Tetracycline	$	D	PS	U / R, B, F
Ticarcillin/clavulanate	$$$$$	B	PS	H / R, B
Tmp/smx	$	D	U	H / R, F
Tobramycin	$$$$	D	U	N / R
Valacyclovir	$$$$$	B	PS	G, H, I / F, R
Valganciclovir	$$$$$	C	N	G, H, I / R
Vancomycin	$$$$$	C	U	N / R (IV), F (oral)
Voriconazole	$$$$$	D	U	H / R
Zalcitabine	_	C	N	I/ R
Zanamivir	$$$$$	C	U	N / R

LEGEND

Metabolism/Excretion

R – Renal
B – Bile
H – Hepatic
F – Feces
O – Other
U – Unknown
S – Sweat
N – None
I – Intracellular
G – GI

Pregnancy Categories

A – Controlled human studies show no risk
B – Animal studies show no risk of adverse fetal effects, but human studies unavailable
C – Animal studies show adverse fetal effects, but no controlled human studies
D – Positive evidence of human fetal risk; maternal benefit may outweigh fetal risk
X – Contraindicated: Positive evidence of serious fetal abnormalities in humans

Cost

$ = <$25
$$ = $25–$49
$$$ = $50–$99
$$$$ = $100–$199
$$$$$ = >$200

Lactation Safety

S – Safe
N – Not Safe
PS – Probably Safe
PN – Probably Not Safe
U – Unknown

IDEAL BODY WEIGHT CALCULATOR

Males		
Height (in)	Height (cm)	Ideal body weight (kg)
60	152.4	50
61	154.94	52
62	157.48	55
63	160.02	57
64	162.56	59
65	165.1	62
66	167.64	64
67	170.18	66
68	172.72	68
69	175.26	71
70	177.8	73
71	180.34	75
72	182.88	78
73	185.42	80
74	187.96	82
75	190.5	85
76	193.04	87
77	195.58	89
78	198.12	91
79	200.66	94
80	203.2	96

Females		
Height (in)	Height (cm)	Ideal body weight (kg)
60	152.4	46
61	154.94	48
62	157.48	50
63	160.02	52
64	162.56	55
65	165.1	57
66	167.64	59
67	170.18	62
68	172.72	64
69	175.26	66
70	177.8	69
71	180.34	71
72	182.88	73
73	185.42	75
74	187.96	78
75	190.5	80
76	193.04	82
77	195.58	85
78	198.12	87
79	200.66	89
80	203.2	92

Drugs to consider using IBW: aminoglycosides, acyclovir, colistin, ethambutol, pyrazinamide

Aminoglycoside dosing weight = *ideal* body weight (IBW); if *actual* body weight (ABW) <IBW dosing weight = ABW; if morbidly obese (>20% over *ideal* body weight) dosing weight = adjusted body weight (AdjBW)

   Males: IBW = 50 kg + 2.3 kg for each inch over 60 inches
   Females: IBW = 45.5 kg + 2.3 kg for each inch over 60 inches
   AdjBW = 0.4 (ABW–IBW) + IBW

COMMON PEDIATRIC ANTIBIOTIC DOSING

Approximate Pediatric Antibiotic Dosing		Weight by Kgs									
Medication (per dose)	Strength (t=5ml)	Freq	5	6.5	8	9	10	11	13	15	19
Amoxicillin (high dose: 40–45 mg/kg)	200/t	2x/day	1	1 ¼	1 ¾	2	2	2 ¼	2 ¾	3	4
	250/t	2x/day	¾	1 ¼	1 ½	1 ½	1 ¾	1 ¾	2 ¼	2 ½	3 ¼
	400/t	2x/day	½	¾	¾	1	1	1 ¼	1 ¼	1 ½	2
Amoxicillin/clavulanate or amoxicillin (25 mg/kg)	125/t	2x/day	1	1 ¼	1 ½	1 ¾	1 ¾	2	2 ¼	2 ¾	3 ½
	200/t	2x/day	½	¾	1	1	1 ¼	1 ¼	1 ½	1 ¾	2 ¼
	250/t	2x/day	½	½	¾	¾	1	1	1 ¼	1 ¼	1 ¾
	400/t	2x/day	¼	½	½	½	¾	¾	¾	1	1
Amoxicillin/clavulanate ES (45 mg/kg)	600/t	2x/day	3/8	½	½	¾	¾	¾	1	1 ¼	1 ½
Azithromycin (5 mg/kg) (5 day course - double dose on day 1)	100/t	daily	–	–	½	½	½	½	¾	¾	1
	200/t	daily	–	–	¼	¼	¼	¼	1/3	½	½
Cefaclor (15–20 mg/kg)	125/t	2x/day	¾	1	1 ¼	1 ½	1 ½	1 ¾	2	2 ½	3
	250/t	2x/day	¼	1/3	¾	¾	¾	1	1	1 ¼	1 ½
Cefdinir (15 mg/kg)	125/t	daily	–	–	1	1	1	1 ¼	1 ½	1 ¾	2
Cefixime (8 mg/kg)	100/t	daily	½	½	¾	¾	¾	1	1	1 ¼	1 ½
Cefuroxime (10–15 mg/kg)	125/t	2x/day	–	¾	¾	1	1	1	1 ½	1 ¾	2 ¼
Cephalexin (10–15 mg/kg)	125/t	4x/day	–	½	¾	¾	1	1	1 ¼	1 ½	1 ¾
	250/t	4x/day	–	¼	¼	½	½	½	¾	¾	1
Nitrofurantoin (1–2 mg/kg)	25/t	4x/day	¼	½	½	½	½	¾	¾	¾	1
TMP/SMX (4 mg/kg)	40/200/t	2x/day	½	¾	1	1	1	1 ¼	1 ½	1 ½	2

*Please note: The dosing is an approximation, with quantities rounded to common non-metric household measurements.

PENICILLIN/CEPHALOSPORIN ALLERGY ALGORITHM FOR ANTIMICROBIAL TREATMENT

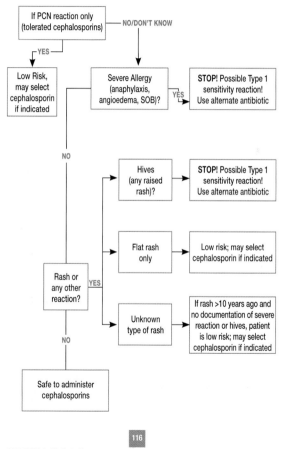

If PCN reaction only (tolerated cephalosporins) → **NO/DON'T KNOW**

YES →

Low Risk, may select cephalosporin if indicated

Severe Allergy (anaphylaxis, angioedema, SOB)? → **YES** → **STOP!** Possible Type 1 sensitivity reaction! Use alternate antibiotic

NO

Rash or any other reaction? → **YES** →

Hives (any raised rash)? → **STOP!** Possible Type 1 sensitivity reaction! Use alternate antibiotic

Flat rash only → Low risk; may select cephalosporin if indicated

Unknown type of rash → If rash >10 years ago and no documentation of severe reaction or hives, patient is low risk; may select cephalosporin if indicated

NO

Safe to administer cephalosporins

ANTIBIOTIC COVERAGE TABLE

	Gram-Positive	Gram-Negative	Anaerobe	Pseudomonas	MRSA	Atypical Bacteria
Penicillin	+		+/-			
Oxacillin	+					
Ampicillin, amoxicillin	+					
Amoxicillin/clavulanate, Ampicillin/sulbactam	+	+	+			
Piperacillin/tazobactam	+	+	+	+		
Ertapenem	+	+	+			
Imipenem	+	+	+	+		
Aztreonam		+		+		
Ciprofloxacin	+	+		+		+
Moxifloxacin	+	+	+			+
Levofloxacin	+	+		+		+
Cefazolin, cephalexin	+	+				
Cefoxitin, cefotetan	+	+	+			
Ceftriaxone	+	+				
Cefepime	+	+		+		
Gentamicin		+		+		
Clindamycin	+		+		+	
Vancomycin	+				+	
TMP/SMX	+	+			+	
Tetracyclines	+	+			+	+
Linezolid	+				+	
Metronidazole			+			
Azithromycin	+/-					+

117

INDEX

2015 EMRA Antibiotic Guide

NOTES